FRUITS AND VEGETABLES AS NUTRACEUTICAL

[NATURE'S MEDICINE]

Cognizing the significance of fruits and vegetables in the human diet. This book is designed to provide an insight into the nutritional importance of fruits and vegetables in human health, disease prevention, managing stress and boosting immunity, especially in this COVID-19 pandemic.

The book contains a very concise and precise information on nutraceuticals, their sources and benefits. It also contains the best possible information regarding common health issues faced by humans and their prevention with the help of bioactive compounds, maintaining a focus throughout on how nutraceuticals influence human health.

The information provided in this book is truly based on scientific records of scientists working in the arena of bioactive compounds of fruits and vegetables and their role in disease prevention of humans as well as Food Safety and Standards Authority of India (FSSAI) acts and regulations.

Mr. Vivek Anumala is presently pursuing his Ph D. in Vegetable Sciences from the College of Horticulture and Forestry, Central Agricultural University, Pasighat, Arunachal Pradesh. He has great enthusiasm in the research of nutraceutical of vegetables and fruits and their importance in health of human beings. He has keen interest in working out the various nutraceutical compounds of Vegetables and Fruits. In future he would like to carry on the recent work on nutraceutical of vegetables and fruits.

Dr. Arunkumar Phurailatpam is currently working as an Associate Professor in Medicinal and Aromatic Plants, College of Horticulture and Forestry, Central Agricultural University, Pasighat, Arunachal Pradesh. He has been working in the field of Medicinal plants and the bioactive contents of various MAPs and Vegetable- fruits.

Dr. Pranabjyoti Sarma is working as an Associate Professor and Head in Vegetable Sciences, College of Horticulture and Forestry, Central Agricultural University, Pasighat, Arunachal Pradesh. He has great knowledge in the cultivation and nutritional values of Vegetables.

FRUITS AND VEGETABLES AS NUTRACEUTICAL

[NATURE'S MEDICINE]

VIVEK ANUMALA
ARUNKUMAR PHURAILATPAM
and
PRANABJYOTI SARMA

NARENDRA PUBLISHING HOUSE
DELHI (INDIA)

First published 2022
by CRC Press
2 Park Square, Milton Park, Abingdon, Oxon, OX14 4RN

and by CRC Press
6000 Broken Sound Parkway NW, Suite 300, Boca Raton, FL 33487-2742

CRC Press is an imprint of Informa UK Limited

British Library Cataloguing-in-Publication Data
A catalogue record for this book is available from the British Library

Library of Congress Cataloging-in-Publication Data
A catalog record has been requested

ISBN: 978-1-032-13800-8 (hbk)
ISBN: 978-1-003-23088-5 (ebk)

DOI: 10.1201/9781003230885

MIX
Paper from responsible sources
FSC™ C013985
FSC www.fsc.org

Printed in the United Kingdom
by Henry Ling Limited

CONTENTS

PREFACE

In this pandemic, realizing the criticality of fruits and vegetables, their role in human health and boosting immunity as nutraceuticals. This book is embellished as a ready reckoner for maintaining daily health of an individual.

This book is crafted diligently to articulate the research advances in the field of "Nutraceuticals" at global level. Further, this book is inclusive of basics which makes this book worth reading. Since knowledge is ocean and has never ending horizon, we exerted our best efforts to compile best available information in this domain.

The information furnished is accumulated from research articles of authentic journals, books, manuals, Indian gazette, regulations, Indian acts and other hand books. We are happy that this book may be useful for UG, PG, Ph.D. students, teachers and other people who love learning horticulture, food technology and dietetics.

A book without an error is not a book

.....Anonymous

Every attempt has been made to present this book error free and we solely take the responsibility of any lack and error. Further, we will be glad welcoming our readers to suggest (anumala.vivek@gmail.com) the improvements and corrections if any, for improving this book. We are extremely thankful to our teachers for their wisdom.

We wish you for good health.

Authors

CHAPTER 1

INTRODUCTION

Food concept has altered significantly over time and the transition from a primitive form of human (*Homo erectus*) to civilised human (*Homo sapiens*) has a significant impact on the nutritional security of humankind. Globalisation entangled humankind among the choices of the right kind of food for his proper growth and development. The lifestyle adopted by the people today has modified the essential food habits of the latter. Consumption of junk food has inflated, resulting in a variety of diseases caused due to improper nutrition. Obesity is a global issue now. Heart disease is still a cause of death in the majority of the nations followed by cancer, obesity, osteoporosis, obesity, arthritis and several more. Malnutrition cost of the world is about 3.5 trillion USD per year (FAO). Consumers being embarrassed with the expensive, high-tech, disease-treatment approach in the modern medicines are seeking complementary or alternative beneficial products and the procedure of managed care makes nutraceutical significantly appealing (Das *et al.*, 2011). "Let food be thy medicine and medicine be thy food", quoted by Hippocrates about 2,500 years ago is undoubtedly the tenet of today. Nutraceuticals are the emerging class of natural products with great potential that make the line between food and drugs to fade (Adelaja and Schilling, 1999). Ayurveda, one of the world's oldest medical systems, promoted the use of herbal compounds in the health care system (Rajasekaran *et al.*, 2008). Mother Nature has conferred humanity with numerous plant species having medicinal properties, untapped till date. Fruits are an excellent source of minerals, vitamins, antioxidants, anti-inflammatory and anti-microbial phytochemicals (Goff and Klee, 2006). Fruits and vegetables have immense potential of being developed into nutritional ingredients and supplements which have changed the perception of horticultural crops and products (Hui *et al.*, 2010; Kalra, 2003). The exploitation of fruits and vegetables is though in its aborning stage, though soon production of nutraceuticals on a large scale could be a reality with the advancement of science and technology.

CHAPTER 2

PRESENT SCENARIO OF NUTRACEUTICAL MARKET

The demand for nutraceuticals as well as functional foods is expected to witness a surge because of consumers opting for immunity-boosting nutritional supplements during the COVID-19 pandemic. A decline in the use of seafood, meat and poultry products across the globe is expected to raise the need for plant-based protein supplements in the future. According to business wire report, global nutraceutical market is expected to cross USD 722.49 billion by 2027 from the level of $182.6 billion (2016), growing at compound annual growth rate (CAGR) of about 8.3%. India's rich heritage of herbal medicines and supplements has found resonance in our mythology and folklore. Due to awareness about fitness, wellness and altering lifestyles, India's nutraceutical market is likely to cross $18 billion by 2025 from the current level of $4 billion (2017) growing at compound annual growth rate (CAGR) of about 17%, according to a study on 'The growing nutraceuticals market in India', conducted by Invest India.

CHAPTER 3

FOOD AND NUTRIENT INTAKE BEHAVIOUR OF INDIANS

In Indian 380 million population are undernourished. While the calorie sufficient but nutrient-deficient population stands at 570 million (NSSO). In a report given by NIN during the year 2015-16 the intake of green leafy vegetables (GLV), milk and milk products and sugar and jaggery were lower than the suggested level of ICMR in an Indian population. The intake of all nutrients is lower than that suggested by the Indian Council of Medical Research.

1. FOOD CONSUMPTION

The average intake of cereals and millets is 320 g/CU/day, while the intake of pulses and legumes is 42 g/CU/day, which is on par with the levels suggested by ICMR (Fig. 1).

2. NUTRIENTS INTAKE

The average intake of the macronutrients such as energy and protein and micronutrients like iron, thiamine and niacin are below the RDA (Fig. 2), whereas, the intake of vitamin A and riboflavin is grossly inadequate. Intake of vitamin C and total folic acid are meeting the RDA (NIN). The proportion

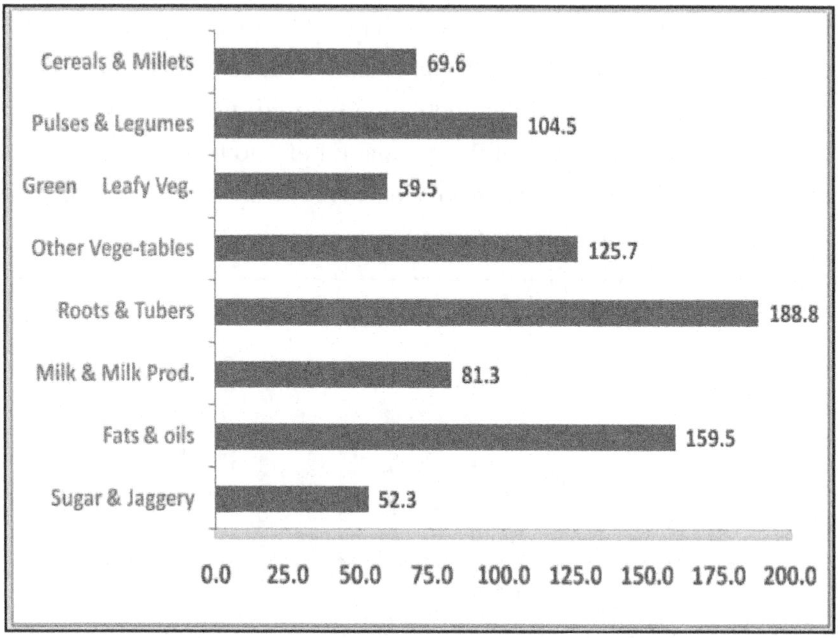

Fig. 1. Food consumption pattern in India
Source: ICMR

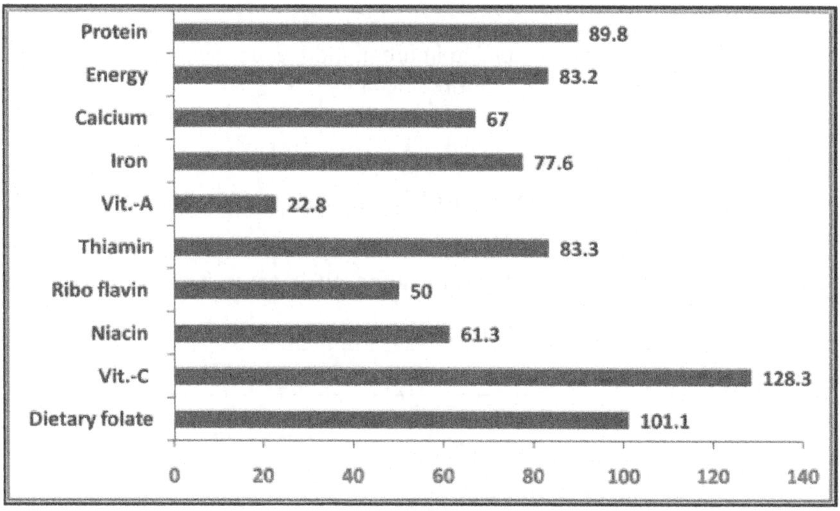

Fig. 2. Nutrient intake pattern in India
Source: ICMR

of preschool children consuming less than 50% of RDA of vitamins and minerals such as vitamin A, riboflavin, vitamin C, dietary folate and calcium is very high. Only 56% of the population who fall in the age bracket of 1–3 years, two-third (68%) of the population of 4 to 6 years old children and half of the population of pregnant women (56%) are consuming adequate amounts of both protein and calories.

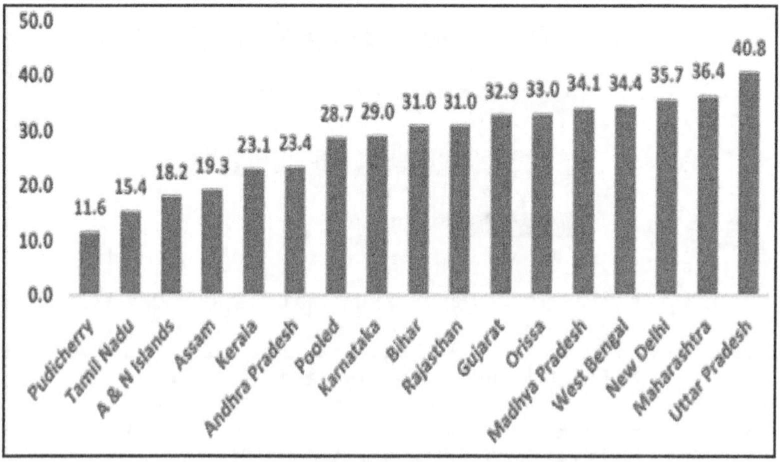

Fig. 3. Prevalence(%) of stunting in urban India under five-year children
Source: ICMR

However, the prevalence of undernutrition (thinness) is significantly higher in 6 to 11 years old and 12 to 17 years old boys as compared to girls of the same age group (Fig. 4).

Table 1. Recommended Dietary Allowance (RDA) table for an Average Man doing Moderate work

Nutrient	RDA
Protein (g)	60
Total Fat (g) (visible + invisible)	30+30
Visible fat or oil(g)	30

[Table Contd.

Contd. Table]

Nutrient	RDA
Energy (kcal)	2727
Calcium (mg)	600
Iron (mg)	17.0
Vitamin A (µg)	600
Carotene (µg)	4800
Thiamine (mg)	1.7
Riboflavin (mg)	1.7
Niacin (mg)	18
Pyridoxine (mg)	2.0
Ascorbic acid (vitamin C) (mg)	40
Folic Acid (µg) (free/Total)	200
Vitamin B12 (µg)	1.0
Magnesium (mg)	340
Zinc(mg)	12

Source: ICMR

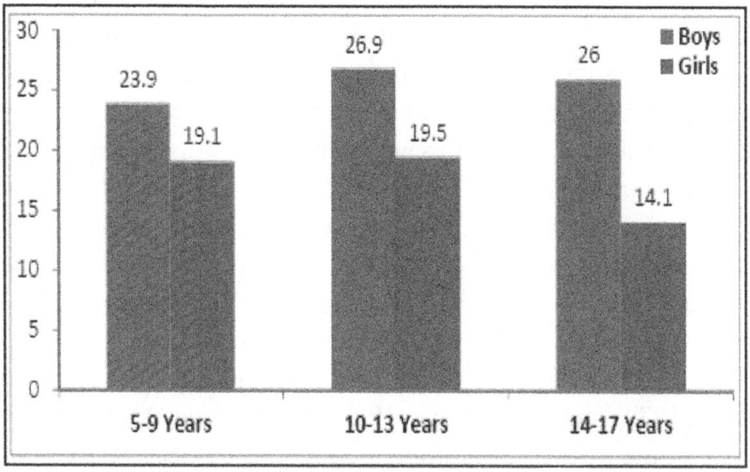

Fig. 4. Prevalence (%) of thinness among school-age children and adolescents
Source: ICMR

CHAPTER 4

IMPORTANCE OF NUTRACEUTICALS

Phytochemicals are potent antioxidants which can modify metabolic activity, detoxify carcinogens, and also influence processes in a tumour cell. The consumption of different kinds of fruits and vegetables is advised, rather than limiting oneself to those who have the highest antioxidant capacity (Wargovich, 2000). Human health improves by eating fresh fruits and vegetables comprising compounds such as phytochemicals. For maintaining good health, there is a need of 50 nutrients that fall into six groups: carbohydrates, proteins, lipids, vitamins (Table 2), minerals and water. Segal *et al.* (1983) reported that the primary nutrients are proteins with the essential amino acids, lipids with the corresponding fatty acids, minerals, vegetable fibres and mineral salts. The ratio of the compounds, their quality, availability and usage are more critical as compared to the nutrient material. There is a natural dietetic value for the fruits and vegetables through their significant content in minerals, alimentary fibres, pectic compounds, amino acids, polyunsaturated fatty acids, vitamins, antioxidants (polyphenols, sulphur compounds, resveratrol), phytoncides (natural antibiotics). Favier *et al.* (1995) reported that it must not be regarded as something positive because no exaggeration is well received. Goncea (1970) and Dumitrescu (1987) in their study, noted that about 14-17% of the caloric value of the food ratio is by fruits and vegetables, the maximum ratio for consumption should be 17% by children, pregnant or nurturing women, as well as the workers from polluted or toxic sectors.

The intestinal transit may be troubled by excessive fibre supply if its consumption exceeds by 1.5 kg/day (Dumitrescu, 1987; Goncea, 1970). Reports suggest that optimum consumption of tomatoes and their products helps in carcinogenesis reduction, especially regarding prostate cancer. It may be due to lycopene, which gives tomatoes their red colour (Giovannucci, 2002).

Table 2. Dietary Table showing significant sources of vitamins and their health benefits

Name of vitamin	Source	Health benefits
Vitamin A_1	Fish liver oil, liver	Antioxidants help in the maintenance of skin health, vision and mucous membrane, prevents Night blindness, Xeropthalmia
Vitamin A_2	Cheese, butter, carrots, spinach, pumpkins, papaya, mango, beet leaf, colocasia leaf, fenugreek leaf.	
Vitamin D	Fish liver oil, wheat germ oil, egg yolk, milk, butter	Essential for formation of bones and teeth, it helps the body to absorb and use calcium, prevents Rickets, Pigeon chest in children and Osteomalacia in adults
Vitamin E (Tocopherol)	Wheat germ oil, cottonseed oil, peanut oil	Promotes formation of blood cells, muscles, lung and nerve tissue, boosts the immune system, Prevents Sterility problems
Vitamin K (Phylloquinone)	Cabbage, cauliflower, tomatoes, soybean	Essential for blood coagulation

[Table Contd.

Contd. Table]

Vitamin B_1	Cashew nut, walnut, chillies Cereals, pulses, leafy vegetables	Essential for neurological related activities, it prevents Beriberi (Disturbance in the digestive system)
Vitamin B_2	Bael, papaya, fenugreek leaves, Nuts, yeast	Helps in energy production, it prevents Photophobia, inflamed lips, cracks on skin or ariboflavinosis
Vitamin B_3 (Pantothenic)	Liver, meat, yeast	Aids inthe conversion of food into energy and maintains proper brain function
Folic acid	Green vegetables, green leafy vegetables like palak	Essential During pregnancy helps in RBC formation, and it prevents anaemia
Vitamin B_5 (Nicotinic acid or Niacin or Nicotinamide)	Yeast, egg, milk	Required for various nervous system function, it prevents Pellagra or black tongue
Vitamin B_6 (Pyridoxine)	Banana, Tomato juice, wheat germ, legumes	Aids inthe production of essential proteins and their conversion into energy, it prevents degeneration of nerves
Biotin (Vitamin H)	Swiss chard	Required for various metabolic functions, prevents Dermatitis
Vitamin B_{12} (Cyanocobalamin)	Animal food like liver, meat, fish, egg	It prevents Pernicious anaemia
Vitamin C	Aonla, guava, citrus fruits	The best antioxidant that prevents Scurvy

Source: Chauhan *et al.*, 2013

CHAPTER 5

NUTRACEUTICAL: DEFINITION AND CONCEPT

The definition of nutraceutical gave by the American Nutraceutical Association, well known for publishing the JANA Journal. Dr Stephen DeFelice, the chairperson of the Foundation for Innovation in Medicine, coined the term "Nutraceutical" is a combination of nutrition and pharmaceutical in 1989. He stated that "A nutraceutical is any substance that is a food or a part of a food and provides medical or health benefits, including the prevention and treatment of disease. Such products may range from isolated nutrients, dietary supplements and specific diets to genetically engineered designer foods, herbal products and processed foods such as cereals, soups and beverages" (DeFelice, 1995). Products isolated or purified from food but which are generally sold in medicinal forms (capsules) but not associated with food are referred to as nutraceuticals (Fig. 5).

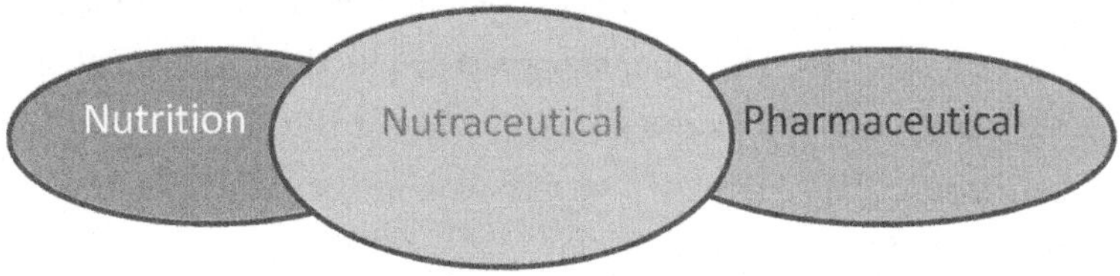

Fig. 5. Linkage of Food, Nutraceutical and Pharmaceutical

The health ministry of Canada defines "Nutraceutical is a product isolated or purified from the food, generally sold in a medicinal form not associated with food and demonstrated to have physiological benefits and also benefits against chronic diseases" (Pandey *et al.*, 2010). It refers to the bioactive components that arepresent in (a) Normal foods, (b) Enriched foods (Functional food) and (c) Dietary supplements, the term nutraceutical is commonly used in marketingunder American legislation and has no regulatory definition. According tothe alteration made by Health Canada, which defines nutraceutical as, "a product isolated or purified from foods, and generally sold in medicinal forms not usually associated with food and demonstrated to have a physiological benefit or provide protection against chronic disease" (Wilkerson *et al.,* 2007).

1. FUNCTIONAL FOOD

It is a frequently used term for any whole food product which contains nutraceuticals (Fig. 6). It plays a vital role in the prevention of chronic diseases (Liu, 2003), as it contains a significant amount of bioactive components which provides desirable health benefits supplementing essential nutrition. In general, the consumption of functional foods is as part of a regular diet which delivers numerous active ingredients which enhance health and also have physiological effects within the food matrix. This confusion is clarified by (González-Sarrías *et al.,* 2013) by differentiating functional foods, nutraceuticals, medical foods, and botanicals. Functional foods provide specific health benefits beyond their nutritional format, which are scientifically proven. They include processed foods or foods with health-promoting additives such as the addition Bio-fortification of cauliflower with β-carotene.

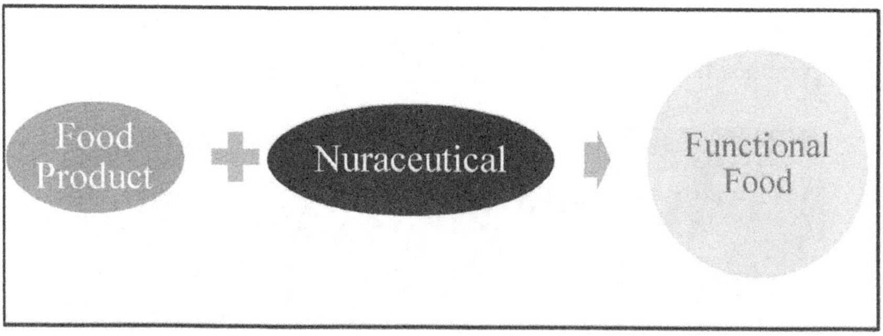

Fig. 6. Functional food

Examples:

(a) Yoghurt - Acts as Probiotics for intestinal health, it is a food produced by bacterial fermentation of milk.

(b) Foods/cereals/snacks enriched with soluble fibre, vitamins, minerals.

(c) Cholesterol - lowering spreads containing phytosterols (Arnoldi, 2010).

2. DIETARY (OR FOOD) SUPPLEMENTS

These are the products that are meant for consumption comprising of a dietary ingredient, to add further nutrition by supplementing the natural diet. Fatty acids, vitamins, minerals, amino acids, or fibre is included, besides other substances. There are more than 50,000 dietary supplements which are mostly multivitamins. The Dietary supplements are generally consumed in a pharmaceutical format i.e., pill, tablet, powder but not as beverages (soups, juices) or conventional foods.

3. ANTIOXIDANT PLANT PIGMENTS

Primarily carotenoids and flavonoids are referred to as phytochemicals. Phytochemical is a broad term and used for a variety of compounds produced by plants like Allyl propyl disulfides, anthocyanins, catechins, carotenoids, flavonoids, flavones, isoflavones, isothiocyanates, phytonutrients, and polyphenols. Findings reveal that there are about 4000 phytochemicals found in vegetables, fruit, beans, and grains (González-Sarrías *et al.*, 2013).

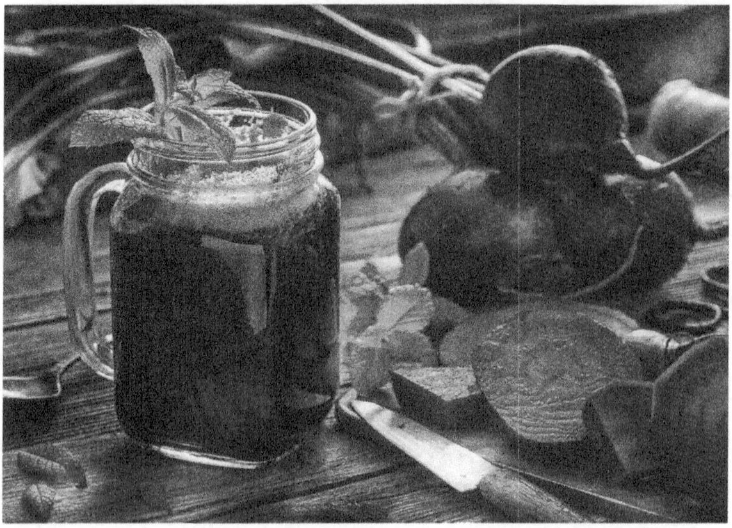

Fig. 7. Beetroot rich in betalains

CHAPTER 6

DIFFERENCE BETWEEN PHARMACEUTICAL AND NUTRACEUTICAL

There is considerable confusion regarding the terminologies like nutraceuticals, functional foods, dietary supplements, designer foods, medical foods, pharmafoods and phytochemicals. However, there seems to be a difference in their interchangeable usage by different people on different occasions. The drugs mainly used to treat diseases are referred to as "Pharmaceuticals" while the drugs which prevent diseases are called "Nutraceuticals" (Rajasekaran *et al.*, 2008). Origin of many pharmaceuticals is from plants and animals and is no less "natural" than nutrients. Synthetic vitamins are classic examples of nutrients.

Table 3. Pharmaceutical Vs Nutraceutical

Pharmaceutical	Nutraceutical
• Synthetically compounded chemicals that affect physiological functions	• While the chemicals derived from plants, or proteins and vaccines derived from animal sources may have the distinction of being called nutraceuticals
• Manufactured specifically for medical use, under a physician's supervision	• Physician's supervision may not be required

[Table Contd.

Contd. Table]

Pharmaceutical	Nutraceutical
• Subject to food and drugs administration approval	• Health supplements (including nutraceuticals, food or dietary supplements) may do not need any approval
• As per the rules of FDA, prescription or recommendation from a certified medical practitioner is essential for the purchase	• Choice of a health supplement is up to the individual and sold without restrictions at health food stores

CHAPTER 7

FOOD SAFETY AND STANDARDS

The food safety and standards (health supplements, nutraceuticals, food for special dietary use, food for special medical purpose, functional food and novel food) regulations, 2016 has been notified by FSSAI on 23/12/2016. FSSAI defined specific terms and their schedules. Some of them are:

(A) "Foods for special dietary uses or functional foods or nutraceuticals or health supplements" means:

(a) foods which are specially processed or formulated to satisfy particular dietary requirements which exist because of a particular physical or physiological condition or specific diseases and disorders and which are presented as such, wherein the composition of these foodstuffs must differ significantly from the composition of ordinary foods of comparable nature, if such ordinary foods exist, and may contain one or more of the following ingredients, namely:-

(i) plants or botanicals or their parts in the form of powder, concentrate or extract in water, ethyl alcohol or hydroalcoholic extract, single or in combination;

(ii) minerals or vitamins or proteins or metals or their compounds or amino acids (in amounts not exceeding the Recommended Daily Allowance for Indians) or enzymes (within permissible limits);

(iii) substances from the animal origin;

(iv) a dietary substance for use by human beings to supplement the diet by increasing the total dietary intake;

(b) **(i)** a product that is labelled as a "Food for special dietary uses or functional foods or nutraceuticals or health supplements or similar such foods" which is not represented for use as a conventional food and whereby such products may be formulated in the form of powders, granules, tablets, capsules, liquids, jelly and other dosage forms but not parenteral, and are meant for oral administration;

(ii) such product does not include a drug as defined in clause (b) and ayurvedic, sidha and unani drugs as defined in clauses (a) and (h) of section 3 of the Drugs and Cosmetics Act, 1940 (23 of 1940) and rules made thereunder;

(iii) does not claim to cure or mitigate any specific disease, disorder or condition (except for particular health benefit or such promotion claims) as may be permitted by the regulations made under this Act;

(iv) does not include a narcotic drug or a psychotropic substance as defined in the Schedule of the Narcotic Drugs and Psychotropic Substances Act, 1985 (61 of 1985) and rules made thereunder and substances listed in Schedules E and EI of the Drugs and Cosmetics Rules, 1945;

(B) "Food for special medical purpose" means food intended for:

(i) particular dietary use specially processed or formulated;

(ii) the dietary management of persons and used only under medical advice;

(iii) the exclusive or partial feeding of persons with a limited, impaired or disturbed capacity to take, digest, absorb, metabolise or excrete ordinary foodstuffs or certain nutrients contained therein or metabolites; or

(iv) other medically determined nutrient requirements, whose dietary management cannot be achieved only by modification of the regular diet, by food for specific nutritional use, or a combination of them;

(C) **"Food with added prebiotic ingredients"** means food that contains added prebiotic ingredients which are non-viable food components that confer health benefits to the consumer by modulation of gut microbiota;

(D) **"Food with added probiotic ingredients"** means food with live micro-organisms beneficial to human health, which when ingested in adequate numbers as a single strain or as a combination of cultures, confer one or more specified or demonstrated health benefits in human beings;

(E) **"Novel food"** means an article of food for which standards have not been specified but is not unsafe: Provided that such food does not contain any of the foods and ingredients prohibited under this Act and regulations made thereunder;

(F) **"Nutritional ingredients"** means the ingredients specified in Schedules other than the food additives specified in Schedule VA to Schedule VF, packed and made available in a form, not for retail-consumer use, but meant for use in formulating a product falling under various categories of these regulations or other categories specified in the Food Safety and Standards (Food Products Standards and Food Additives) Regulations, 2011;

(G) **"Pre-mixes"** means a combination of two or more ingredients specified in the Schedules in a specific proportion with or without additives, packed and meant for use in formulating a product falling under any category of these regulations or under the categories specified in the Food Safety and Standards (Food Products Standards and Food Additives) Regulations, 2011;

(H) **"Specialty food containing plant or botanical ingredients"** means food which is shown to be containing plant or botanical ingredients with a history of safe usage.

(I) "Nutraceuticals"- The nutraceuticals shall provide a physiological benefit and help maintain good health.

(i) A food business operator may extract, isolate and purify nutraceuticals from food or non-food sources, that is preparing amino acids and their derivatives by bacterial fermentation under controlled conditions.

(ii) The nutraceuticals shall contain any of the ingredients specified in Schedule I or Schedule II or Schedule IV or Schedule VI or Schedule VII or Schedule VIII.

(iii) No ingredient other than those specified in Schedule VI shall be used as nutraceutical with standardisation to marker compounds specified and at daily usage levels specified therein.

(iv) No food business operator shall use the extract of the ingredient as nutraceutical other than that specified in Schedule IV Provided that the ingredient of plant or botanical origin specified in Schedule IV and Schedule VI may be used either in the given form, or their extract, subject to the extractive ratios concerning the daily usage value.

(v) No food business operator shall use additives for nutraceutical formulation except those specified in Schedule VA or Schedule VE or Schedule VF.

(J) "Health supplements"- Health supplements may be used to supplement the regular diet of a person above the age of five years.

(i) The health supplements shall contain any of the ingredients specified in Schedule I or Schedule II or Schedule IV or Schedule VII or Schedule VIII or enzymes only of Schedule VI (given ate the end end).

(ii) The health supplements shall contain concentrated source of one or more nutrients, namely, amino acids, enzymes, minerals, proteins, vitamins, other dietary substances, plants or botanicals, prebiotics, probiotics and substances from animal origin or other similar substances with known and established nutritional or beneficial physiological effect, which are presented as such and are offered alone or in combination, but are not drugs as defined in the clause (b) of section 3 of the Drugs and Cosmetics Act, 1940 (23 of 1940) and the rules made thereunder.

(iii) No food business operator shall use additives for health supplement formulation except those specified in Schedule VA **or** Schedule VE or Schedule VF.

(K) Some important highlights of regulations

- Food business operator may use the approved colours and additives permitted in Schedule VF
- Under the regulation four for sub-regulation (1), a nutritional claim shall consist of the 'Ingredients (nutrient or nutritional) content' of an article of food which shall be subject to the nutritional supplement requirements specified in Schedule I, Schedule II, Schedule III, Schedule IV, and Schedule VI.

CHAPTER 8

CLASSIFICATION OF NUTRACEUTICALS

Nutraceuticals are classified in several ways (Chauhan *et al.,* 2013) depending upon understanding and application, i.e. for academic instruction, clinical trial design, functional food development or dietary recommendations. Most common ways to classify nutraceuticals are:

1. **Natural food sources:** It is the classification of the products based on the source obtained from, e.g. plants, animals, minerals or microbial sources.
2. **Mechanism of action:** It generally depends upon how phytochemical behaves and its mode of action:
    (1) A Substrate for biochemical reactions
    (2) Acts as a cofactor of the enzymatic reaction
    (3) Inhibitors of the enzymatic reactions (Fig. 8)
    (4) Absorbents that bind to and eliminate the undesirable constituent in the intestine
    (5) Enhance the absorption or stabilise essential nutrients
    (6) Act as a selective growth factor for beneficial bacteria
    (7) Fermentation substrate for beneficial bacteria
    (8) Act as a selective inhibitor of harmful intestinal bacteria

(9) Function as scavengers of reactive or toxic chemicals

(10) Operate like ligands that antagonise cell surface or intracellular receptors (Chauhan *et al.,* 2013).

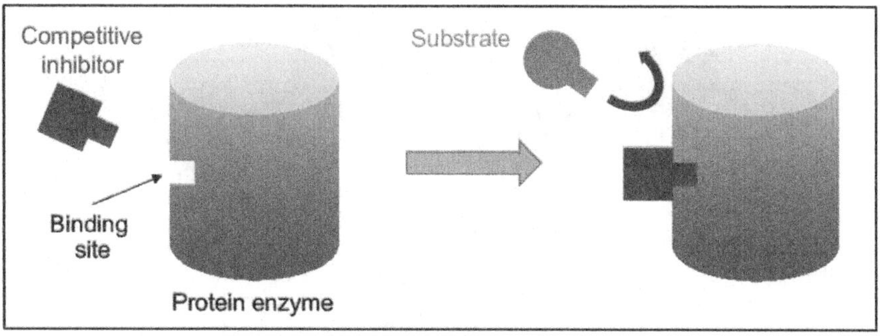

Fig. 8. Inhibition of enzymatic reaction

3. **According to their chemical nature**: Nutraceutical is an inclusive term which includes a variety of compounds which ranges from essential metals, large polymers up to bacteria. The chemical nature of nutraceuticals depends typically on their structure and function. Nutraceuticals categorised under different molecular or elemental groups and subgroups are listed below.

   a. **Amino acid-based substances:** amino acids (Fig. 9), ally-S compounds, indole, folate and choline

   b. **Carbohydrates and derivatives:** ascorbic acid, oligosaccharides, nonstarch-polysaccharides

   c. **Fatty acids and structural lipids:** lecithin, fatty acids, oil

   d. **Isoprenoid derivatives:** carotenoids, saponins, tocopherols, terpenes

   e. **Phenolic substances:** coumarins, tannins, lignin, anthocyanins, isoflavones, flavones, flavonols

   f. **Microbes:** probiotics, prebiotics

   g. **Minerals:** calcium, selenium, potassium, copper, zinc

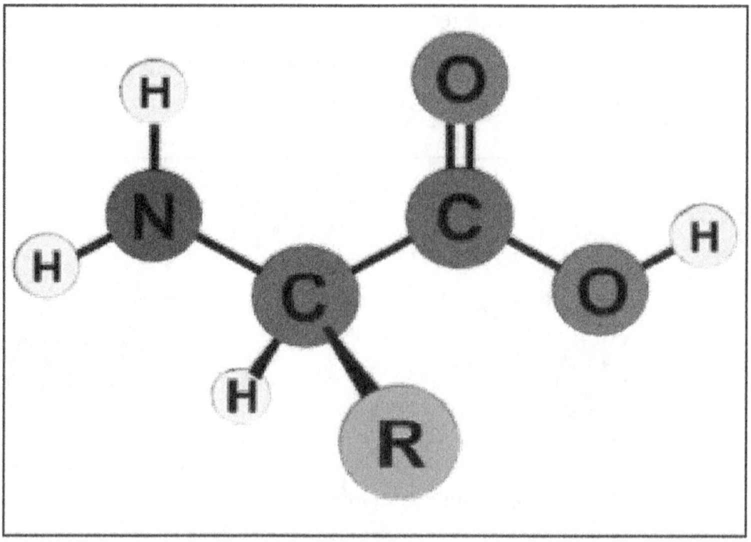

Fig. 9. Alpha-amino acid

More broadly, nutraceuticals are classified into two groups (Pandey *et al.,* 2010).

(a) **Potential Nutraceuticals**: are those who have a promising approach towards particular health or medicinal benefit, and

(b) **Established Nutraceuticals**: A potential nutraceutical can become an established one only after efficient clinical data of its health and medical benefits are obtained and also when there are specific clinical tests available to conduct and demonstrate its results. Reports reveal that many nutraceutical products still fall in the 'potential' category. The food sources used as nutraceuticals are all-natural (Chauhan *et al.,* 2013). The most usual nutraceuticals are nutrients, phytochemicals, dietary supplements, prebiotics, probiotics, functional food and natural herbals chemicals derived from different plant-based sources like fruits, vegetables, medicinal plants are described below (Bickford *et al.,* 2006).

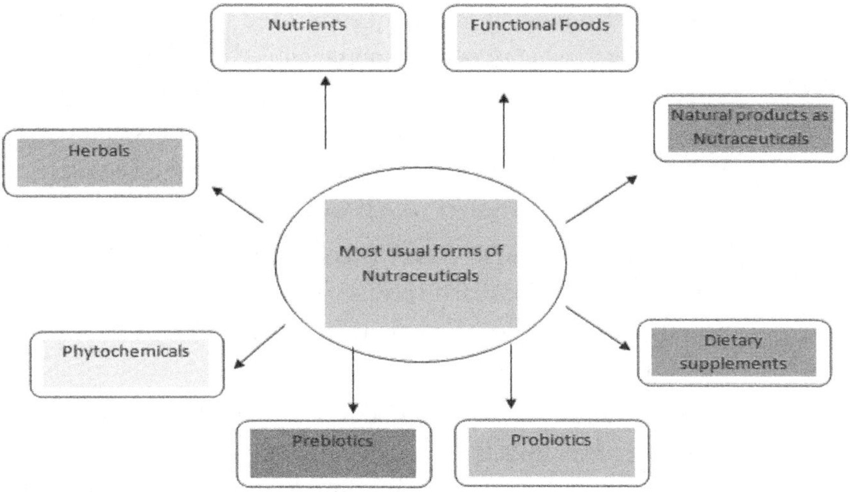

Fig. 10. Different forms of nutraceuticals

1. **Nutrients:** Substances having predefined nutritional functions, such as carbohydrate, proteins, vitamins, minerals, amino acids and fatty acids lie under this category. Antioxidants, vitamins and essential minerals are the most commonly known nutrients. The substances which retard or prevent deterioration, damage or destruction caused by oxidation are known as antioxidants. An integral part of the nutraceutical market is antioxidant (Devi and Rehman, 2002; Sagar *et al.,* 2004). The Phyto-nutrients are the unique substances which occur naturally in plants and have the compelling disease-preventing ability (Sagar *et al.,* 2004; Frasher, 2006; Nordvisk, 1984). Both the essential and nonessential phytonutrients are bioactive food components, based on the specific physiological function they impart, including characterisation of their metabolic and physiological functions and associated targets. Fruits and vegetables provide various essential nutrients which we need: vitamins, minerals, dietary fibre, water, and healthful phytochemicals (Nordvisk, 1984; Trucker, 2003; Sirtori and Galli, 2002).

2. **Functional Foods:** It is a frequently used term for any whole food product which contains nutraceuticals. Functional foods provide specific health benefits beyond their nutritional format, which are proven scientifically. They include processed foods or foods with health-promoting additives such as the addition Bio-fortification of cauliflower with β-carotene.

3. **Natural products as Nutraceuticals:** Almost all the fruits and vegetables have essential minerals which are naturally derived or synthesised, with lower content of fat, calories and no cholesterol (Table 4).

4. **Herbals:** Herbs or botanical products are the natural concentrates or extracts from plants. The medicinal herbs contain numerous nutraceuticals as their principal components (Ravi, 2007; Inti and Faoro, 2006; Shukla and Singh, 2007). These days, attention is more towards the discovery of the link between dietary nutrients and disease prevention. A Large number of herbs play a crucial role in disease prevention. In addition to the macro and micronutrients such as proteins, fats, carbohydrates, vitamins or minerals which are very much essential for a healthy metabolism, a plant-based diet contains numerous non-nutritive phytoconstituents which may also play an essential role in health enhancement (Hamid and Luan, 2000; Mermel, 2004; Dullo *et al.*, 1999; Bell and Goodrick, 2002). The nutraceuticals market comprises two central units: Functional Foods and Dietary Supplements. There is a desperate need for domestication and cultivar development for the cultivation of these plants on a commercial scale. The post-harvest processing technology which allows the material to remain active and hygienic is lacking for the majority of these plants, some of the examples of herbals are *Aloe* vera, Tulsi, Sarpagandha roots, they are used to control or prevent various diseases.

Table 4. List of Fruits and Vegetables rich in essential nutrients

Nutrient	Fruit Sources	Vegetable Sources
Calcium	Litchi, Blackberries, Blackcurrants, Dates, Grapefruit, Mulberries, Orange, Pomegranate	Agathi, Amaranth leaves, Celery, Chinese Broccoli, French Beans, Okra, Spirulina, Turnip
Copper	Avocado, Blackberries, Dates,Guava, Lychee, Mango, Pomegranate	Amaranth leaves, French Beans, Peas, Potatoes, Pumpkin, Spirulina, Sweet Potato
Iodine	Fruits cultivated in iodine-rich soils contain iodine	Vegetables cultivated in iodine-rich soils contain iodine. Eg. Okra
Iron	Blackberries, Karonda, Cherries, Dates, Figs, Grapes, Kiwi, Lychee, Mulberries, Pomegranate, Strawberry, Watermelon	Amaranth leaves, Agathi, French Beans, Peas, Potatoes, Spinach, Turnip
Magnesium	Banana, Blackberries, Blackcurrants, Dates, Guava, Mulberries, Pomegranate, Raspberries, Watermelon	Amaranth leaves, Butternut squash, French Beans, Okra, Peas
Manganese	Banana, Blackberries, Blackcurrants, Blueberries, Grapefruit, Guava, Pomegranate, Raspberries, Strawberry	French Beans, Lima Beans, OkraPeas, Sweet Potato, Potatoes
Phosphorous	Avocado, Dates, Guava, Lychee, Mulberries, Pomegranate, Almonds, Cashew	Amaranth leaves, Brussels Sprouts, Corn, French Beans, Parsnip, Potatoes, Pumpkin
Potassium	Bananas, Cherries, Dates, Grapefruit, Guava, Pomegranate, Watermelon	Amaranth leaves, Bamboo Shoots French Beans, Parsnips, Potatoes, Pumpkin, Sweet Potatoes
Selenium	Bananas, Guava, Litchi, Mango, Pomegranate, Watermelon	Asparagus, French Beans, Lima Beans, Mushrooms, Peas

[Table Contd.

Contd. Table]

Nutrient	Fruit Sources	Vegetable Sources
Sodium	Found in almost all fresh, whole fruits	Sodium occurs naturally in almost all fresh, whole vegetables
Zinc	Blackberries, Dates, Pomegranate, Raspberries	Asparagus, Bamboo Shoots, Corn, French Beans, Okra, Peas, Potatoes, Pumpkin

5. **Dietary supplements:** Reagents derived from other sources (e.g., pyruvate, chondroitin sulfate, steroid hormone precursors) which serve specific functions mainly in sports nutrition, weight-loss supplements, conventionally fortified foods, and meal replacements. Dietary supplements do not treat or cure disease, whereas nutraceuticals are those who help in the prevention or treatment of diseases. They are concentrated form of nutrients or other substances, alone or in combination, and deliver's a nutritional or physiological effect (Bickford *et al.,* 2006; Devi and Rehman, 2002). Besides that, dietary supplements are those products that can be purchased by the consumer without a prescription. In general, antioxidants may also be useful in the prevention of cancer and cerebrovascular diseases (Bell and Goodrick, 2002; Brouns, 2002; Sirtori and Galli, 2002; Bland, 1996). Dietary supplements are not drugs and the main difference is that unlike drugs, they do not have approved therapeutic claims. Dietary supplements may contain vitamins, minerals, herbals, or amino acids. All targeted to supplement an individual's diet. Dietary supplements should not be taken alone as a substitute for any food or medicine.
6. **Phytochemicals:** The naturally occurring biochemical which provide plants with their colour, flavour, smell, and texture and also help to prevent diseases are known as phytochemicals (Dullo *et al.,* 1999; Brouns, 2002; Bland, 1996). These are biologically active natural products, for example:

a) Glucosinolates in cruciferous vegetables,

b) Limonoids in citrus fruits,

c) Lycopene in tomatoes, and

d) Catechins in tea.

Phytochemicals are used as antioxidants with positive health effects (Bagchi, 2006; Ramaa *et al.*, 2006; Whitman, 2001; Burney, 1989). A broad range of phytopharmaceuticals with a claimed hormonal activity can be called "phytoestrogens", recommended for the prevention of prostate or breast cancer. Flavonoids act as antioxidants with anticarcinogenic properties, besides those carotenoids and lycopene acts as a vital source of phytochemicals for human health. Proanthocyanidins are the phytochemical tannins, which detoxify carcinogens and scavenge harmful free radicals. Ellagic acid, a proven anti-carcinogen, is used in alternative medicine and for preventing cancer (Vattem and Shetty, 2005). Ellagic acid is predominantly present in strawberries, cranberries, walnuts, pecans, pomegranates and the best source is red raspberry seeds.

7. **Prebiotics:** Prebiotics are those substances, which reach to the colon in an intact form without getting depleted or digested by the gastric pH and digestive acids respectively. Prebiotics selectively promote the growth of colon probiotic bacteria acting as fertilisers or substrates for these bacteria. Prebiotics is a collective term for non-digestive, but a fermentable dietary carbohydrate that may promote growth selectively for certain bacterial groups or strains residing in the colon like *Bifidobacteria, Lactobacilli* and benefit the human host (Gibson and Roberfroid, 1995). The prebiotic inulin, which is soluble dietary fibres, and also resistant to the digestive enzymes, hence reaches to large intestine or colon mostly intact, where it gets fermented by resistant bacteria (*Lactobacilli*) (Peppelenbosch and Ferreira, 2009).

8. **Probiotics:** are those substances which consist of microorganisms (Fig. 11) or bacteria that are beneficial to the host organism it may

be plant or animal. In general, "Probiotic" is a term commonly used for "Friendly bacteria". Digestive microbes usually come from uncooked fruits, vegetables, and fermented products intake. About four hundred different bacteria are residing live in the human GI tract, among that *lactobacillus acidophilus* is the dominant strain of probiotic fighter (Miller *et al.,* 2003). There are many benefits of using probiotics as nutraceuticals as reported by (Miller, 2003) some of those include:

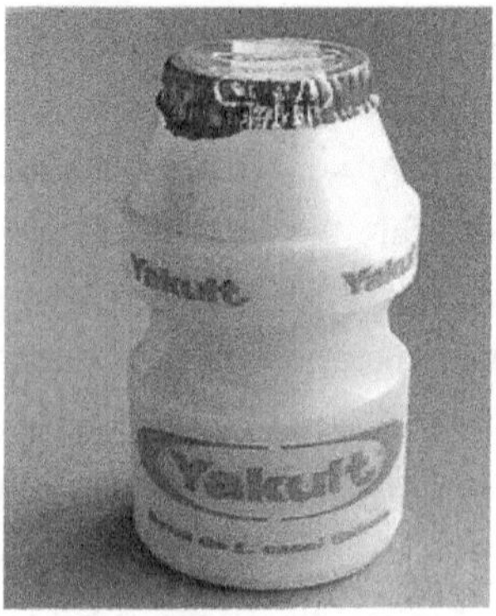

Fig. 11. Probiotic milk

a) Enhancement of bowel function
b) Prevention of colon cancer
c) Lowering cholesterol
d) Lowering of blood pressure
e) Improving immune function
f) Reducing infections
g) Reducing inflammation
h) Improving mineral absorption
i) Preventing the growth of harmful bacteria
j) Fighting off diseases like *Candida* and *Eczema*

CHAPTER 9

BENEFITS OF FRUITS AND VEGETABLES AS NUTRACEUTICALS

Dietary therapeutics or nutraceuticals are used as a complementary therapy in a healing system of nutritional therapy. The basic theory of this therapy is that the foods are not only used as sources of nutrients and energy but also to provide medicinal health benefits. Further, nutraceuticals are also used in detoxifying the body, avoiding vitamin and mineral deficiencies, and restoring healthy digestion and dietary habit. Phytonutrients are plant-derived nutrients with particular biological activities helps in supporting human health (Chauhan *et al.,* 2013).

1. THE NUTRACEUTICAL VALUE

At present many nutraceutical foods are spread (nonalcoholic drinks, spice mixtures, sauces and specially prepared products) which include in their recipes specific components or natural herbs having a medicinal effect namely tonic, stimulative, digestive, protector or antioxidant, which are extracted from the best known and well appreciated cultivated plants or from the spontaneous flora (Dejica, 2001; Florlani *et al.*, 2003; Segal *et al.*, 1986).

Besides, diversity of vegetable products has already entered the human diet and are still entering like nettle and dandelion, as supplements with a supporting role in nourishment viz., vitaminising, stomachic, depurative and sometimes as therapeutic. Due to the lack of appealing texture and relishing taste, people consume them less often. On the contrary, these vegetable products promote overall health. Some examples among vegetables are green leafy vegetables like spinach, and others are garlic, onion, horseradish and broccoli (the entire cabbage family), bell peppers, tomatoes, dill, thyme, ginger and root crops (Table 5), artichoke, peppergrass. Examples among fruits include walnuts, black currants, blackberries, savine and wild roses. The citrus fruits (especially lemons, grapefruit, bitter oranges and bergamots), ginger, turmeric, pimento and papaya are among the tropical products. Red wine, paprika, pepper paste, black currant wine, blackberry products, tomato products, walnut and grape seed oils are various processed products with nutraceutical role in the human diet (Barberan and Robins, 1997).

Table 5. Dietetic, medicinal and alimentary benefits of some major root crops

Species	Main dietetic, medicinal and alimentary features
Carrots	Digestive, hepatic, diuretic, vitaminising, anti-anaemic, depurative, detoxifying and emollient effect; dietetic product for children, sick people or workers in the toxic or radioactive environment
Early radish	Vitaminizing, re-mineralising effect
Radish	Vitaminizing, re-mineralising effect, anti-lithiasis, hepatic and pectoral product. It should be consumed around the year
Beet	Mineralizing, tonic, antibacterial, depurative and diuretic
Celery root	Stimulating agent, general tonic, diuretic, glycaemia reducer; used for winter consumption
Root of parsley	Re-vitalizing, detoxifying effect; aromatising stuff used in the canned food industry and gastronom
Parsnip	Tonic, stomachic, depurative, detoxifying effect

Source: *Beceanu et al., 2008*

The medicinal value is ancillary to the nutraceutical value and one of the possible functions of foodstuff being the therapeutic one and hence some foodstuffs may have medicinal qualities. The entire group of the *Alliaceae* members (garlic, onion, parsnip) synthesise organic compounds like sulphur which intensify or enhance the redox cycle of glutathione and activate specific immunity types (Table 6). Bioactivity of these compounds exhibits an antioxidant, antibacterial, anticarcinogenic, immune-stimulating and liver protective potential. Garlic prevents heart diseases like atherosclerosis, hypercholesterolemia and high blood pressure and cancer. It is an effective remedy against the intestinal Parasites (Olinescu *et al.*, 1990; Picard, 2008; Proust, 2008). Thyme is a selective disinfectant, which is irreplaceable in intestinal infections. There is vast diversity among the species of cabbage, broccoli, heads of cabbage (white, red and savoy), cauliflower and the brussels sprouts have an anti-radical activity proven by their remarkable contents in polyphenols, flavones and condensed tannins. The anthocyanin pigments, especially from black grapes and other coloured fruits, are mainly used in the treatment of many diseases, where the free radicals are involved in the amelioration of the flexibility and reduction of the permeability of capillaries for retina protection (the ocular vascularity). Flavonoids are bioactive substances derived from citrus fruits, tea and wine that have anti-inflammatory activity, fortify the human body against allergies, viruses and the factors inducing tumours.

Table 6. Some of the vital phytochemicals and their action from major horticultural crops

Name	Type of compound	Horticultural Species	Action
Allicin	Sulphur compound	garlic, onion	Bcd, Bst, Fcd, Fst
Tetrahydroallicin	Sulphur compound	onion	Bcd, Bst, Fcd, Fst
Dimethil	Sulphur compound	onion	Bcd, Bst, Fcd, Fst
thiosulfinate			
Tomatidine	Steroidal alkaloid	tomato	Fcd, Fst, (Bst)

[Table Contd.

Contd. Table]

Name	Type of compound	Horticultural Species	Action
Sinigrine	Sulphur glycoside	horseradish, radish, cabbage	Bcd (Bst)
Pinene	Cyclic terpene	mostly fruits and vegetables pigmented in yellow, red, violet or complementary hues	Bst (Bcd)
Derivatives of the cinnamic acid	Phenolic substances		Bst (Bcd)
Derivatives of the benzoic acid	Phenolic substances		Bst (Bcd)
Flavans	Phenolic substances		Bst (Bcd)
Flavones and Isoflavones	Phenolic substances		Bst (Bcd)
Anthocyanin	Phenolic substances		Bst (Bcd)

Bcd=bactericide; Bst=bacterio-static; Fcd=fungicide; Fst=fungi-static

Source: *Beceanu et al., 2008*

Many health problems are related to the digestive system, such as constipation, or the nutrition ones, such as obesity, can be overcome only by adequate nutrition based on fruits and vegetables. The antioxidant effect of carotenoids (β-carotene, lycopene), tocopherols, L-ascorbic acid, polyphenols, capsaicin, resveratrol and other horticultural products can prevent the accelerated ageing, the cardio-vascular and degenerative diseases and many types of cancer (Dumitrescu *et al.*, 1991).

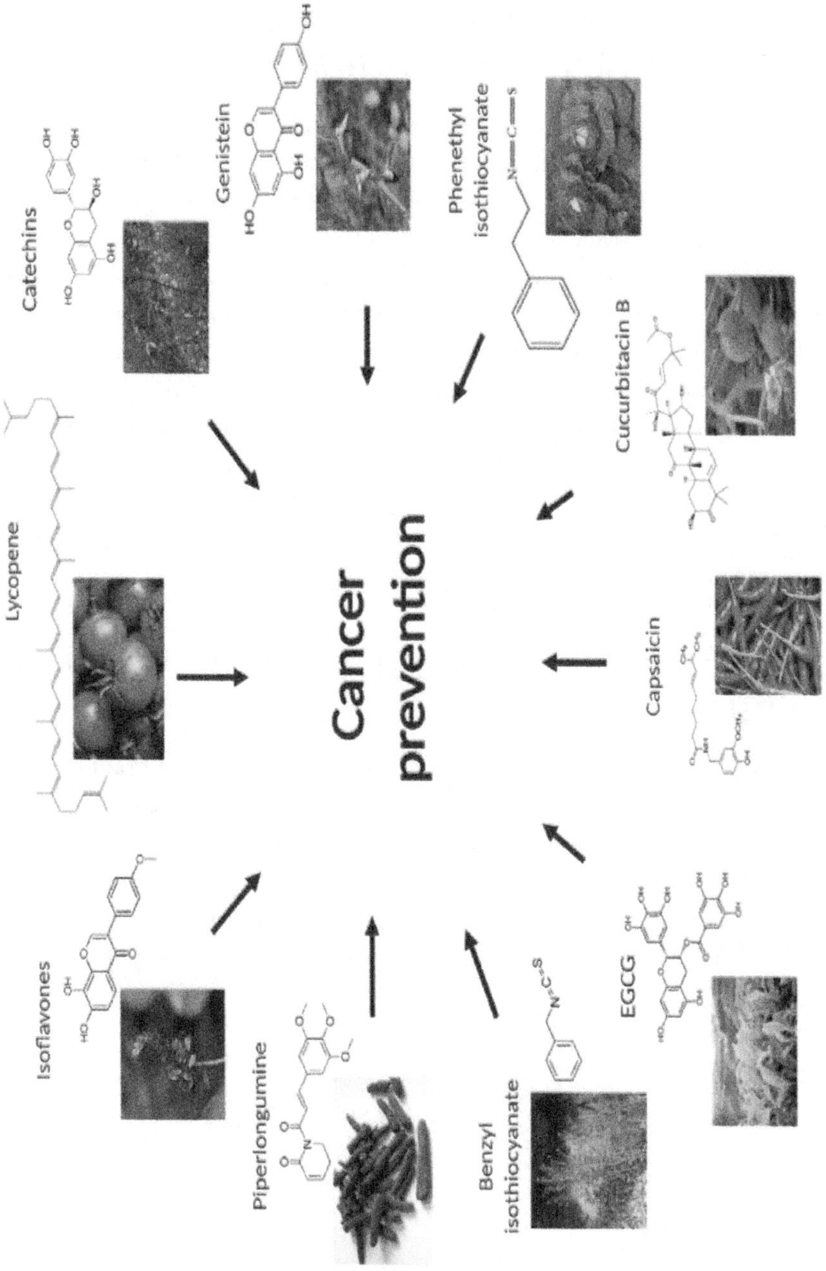

Fig. 12. Different forms of Cancer Preventive Molecules

2. MEDICAL EFFECTS OF NUTRACEUTICAL FRUITS FOR THE COGNITION AND BRAIN HEALTH

Dietary factors influence significantly on specific molecular systems and mechanisms that take care of the mental activity. A diet with a high amount of omega-3 fatty acids is earning accolades for reinforcing cognitive activity in humans (McCann and Ames, 2005) and upregulating genes that are important for sustaining synaptic activity (Wu *et al.*,2007). There is a high risk of many mental disorders, such as attention-deficit disorder, dyslexia, dementia, depression, bipolar disorder, and schizophrenia when humans are deficient in omega-3 fatty acids (Adams *et al.*, 1996; Peet *et al.*, 1996; Hibbeln, 1998; Horobbin, 1998; Freeman *et al.*, 2006). The human body is unable to synthesise omega-3 fatty acid [alpha-linolenic acid (ALA), eicosapentaenoic acid (EPA), and docosahexaenoic acid (DHA)] which are essential for the neuron membranes and that is why we have to depend on our dietary sources.

3. NUTRACEUTICAL FRUITS FOR COGNITION AND BRAIN HEALTH

Fruits and fruit juices are used commonly for cognition and brain health. Kesarvani and Sharma, 2014 found the use of various fruits for brain health because of the medicinal value of fruits, they also reported the role of vitamin C and polyphenols which are found mainly in citrus fruits and blueberries in mental performance. Further nutraceuticals are also helpful for geriatrics. The various phytochemicals found in fruits are listed (Table 7).

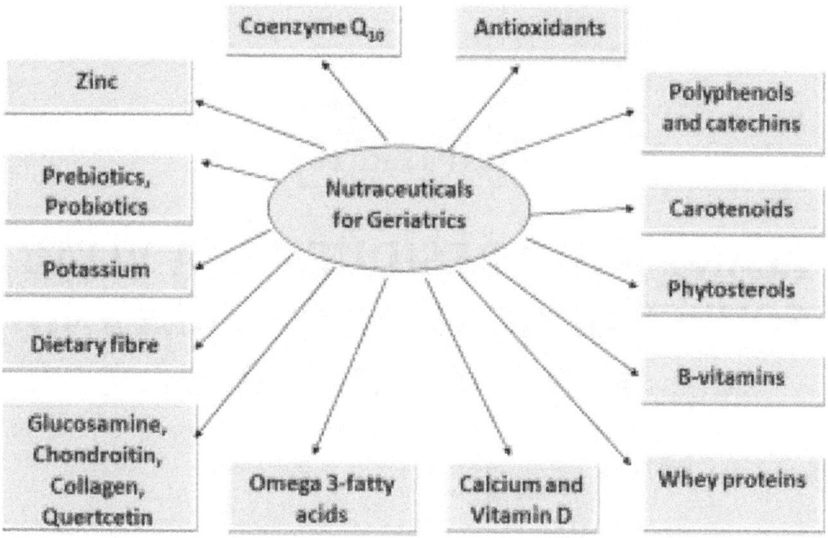

Fig. 13. Nutraceuticals for Geriatrics

Table 7. Major phytochemicals present in fruits

Fruits	Phytochemical compounds
Strawberries	Kaempferol, fisetin, matairesinol, secoisolariciresinol, gallic acid, ellagic acid, and chlorogenic acid
Blackberries	Ellagic acid
Blueberries	Chlorogenic acid, secoisolariciresinol, and pterostilbene
Raspberries	Ellagic Acid, quercetin, gallic acid, cyanidins, pelargonidins, catechins, kaempferol, and salicylic acid
Plum	Lutein, cyanidin
Prunes	Lutein, ursolic acid
Cherries	Limonene
Oranges	Rutin, lutein
Red grapes	Proanthocyanidins
Pomegranates	Ellagitannins, delphinidin, cyanidin, pelargonidin glycosides, catechins, gallocatechin, and prodelphinidins

Source: *Kesarvani and Sharma, 2014.*

CHAPTER 10

PLANT FOOD RESIDUES AS A VITAL SOURCE OF NUTRACEUTICALS AND FUNCTIONAL FOOD

Fruits from the temperate zone are generally characterised by a sizable edible portion and considerable amounts of waste material (peels, seeds and stones) when compared with, significantly higher ratios of by-products arise from tropical and subtropical fruit processing. As a result of increasing production, disposal of the plant material is a massive problem as it is usually prone to microbial spoilage, hampering further exploitation. On the other side, post-processing and handling cost is a limiting factor. Therefore, agro-industrial waste is often utilised as a feed or as fertiliser. Present-day consumers are conscious of diet-related health problems and maintain their diet with the consumption of fruits and vegetables. However, this may not be feasible in every season for everyone. That is why dietary supplements may act as an alternative source to access compounds such as carotenoids, polyphenolics, tocopherols, and vitamin C. Several fruits such as mango, banana, and those belonging to the citrus family creates a massive amount of waste residues in the form of peels, pulp, seeds, and stones. Disposal of these residues is a significant problem due to a lack of infrastructure to handle that much quantities of available biomass, a lack of processing facilities, and high processing costs, high operational cost, especially in developing countries. The total phenolic compounds of seeds as a by-product of fruits, such as mangos, longans, avocados, and jackfruits are higher than that of the total edible product (Soong *et al.*, 2004). The peels and seeds of tomatoes are more abundant sources of phenolic compounds compared to their pulp.

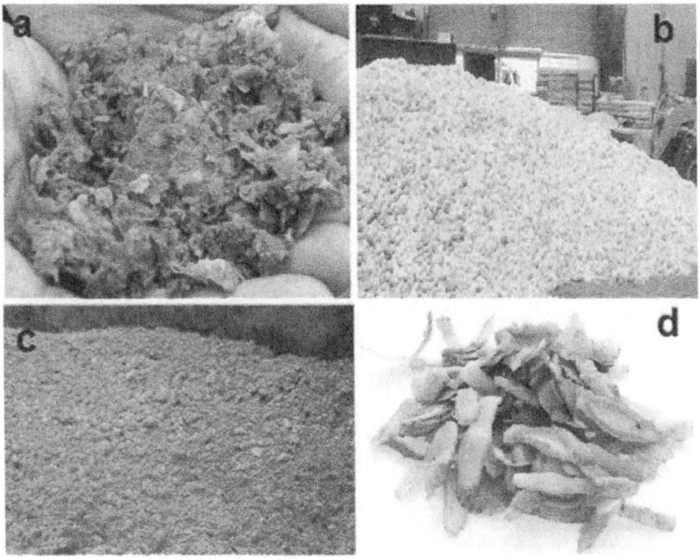

Fig. 14. Some major food wastes: (a). Apple Pomace (b). Lemon Residues (c). Tomato Peels (d). Potato

1. USE OF PLANT FOOD RESIDUES AS A SOURCE FOR FUNCTIONAL FOODS—PHYTOCHEMICALS PRESENCE

Plant metabolites like flavonoids belong to the group of polyphenolics in the human diet, further subdivided into several other groups like flavone, flavonol, flavanone, and isoflavones, these plant polyphenols provide essential health benefits like prevention of metabolic syndrome, cancer, maintains brain health, immune system and overall wellbeing. The phytochemicals like naringin and naringenin are the important citrus flavonoids and aids to control the abnormalities like atherosclerosis (Lee *et al.*, 2001). Besides, bioflavonoids such as hesperidin (from the orange peel), naringin (grapefruit peel) and rutin are reported to have an ability to normalise capillary permeability and vascular brittleness. Hence, they are called vitamin P factors catechins, proanthocyanidins (grapes origin flavanols), e.g. comprises the phenolic compounds of the wine, have which have beneficial effects exerted by moderate consumption of wine (Shrikhande, 2000). Grape seeds are a significant source of proanthocyanidins and can be used for fortifying numerous food products. Grape seed proanthocyanidin extract can neutralise free radicals, protect the over-oxidative damage (Feng and Chen, 2003; Spranger *et al.*, 2008) and lower the incidence of problems caused by free radicals, which includes myocardial infarction, atherosclerosis and drug-induced liver as well as kidney injury. More than that, they are reported to have antithrombotic, antitumor, antimutagenic, anti-radiation-damage, and antifatigue effects (Sano *et al.*, 2005; Engelbrecht *et al.*, 2007). Flavonoids are found in vegetables abundantly. Onion bulbs (*Allium cepa* L.) are the richest sources of dietary flavonoids and contribute to a large portion of the overall consumption of flavonoids. Flavonoids have positive effects on inflammation, cardiovascular diseases, and cancer (Okamoto, 2005). Slimestad *et al.* (2007), reported more than 50 flavonoids in the pigmented scales of onion. Flavonols are the main flavonoids of the pigmented scales of onions and the main flavonols are based on quercetin (3, 5, 7, 30, 40-pentahydroxyflavone). Anthocyanins, carotenoids, betalains, lycopene, and leucoanthocyanidin are the major groups of coloured phenolic compounds in the residues of fruit and vegetable (Table 8). They are effective antioxidants with many pharmacological properties, making them more attractive as "functional foods" for health. On average, two lakh tons of red beet is produced in Western Europe annually for vegetable purpose. The remained portion is processed into juice, colouring foodstuff, and food colourant. Juice industry generates 15%–30% of the pomace from the raw material and though it is still rich in betalains, used as a feed or manure. Betacyanins and betaxanthins are responsible for the vibrant red colour of a beet.

Table 8. Various Phenolic compounds as nutraceuticals from different fruit residues

Fruit	Waste Residue	Phenolic Constituent
Apple	Peel and pomace	Epicatechin, catechins, hydroxycinnamates, phloretin glycosides, quercetin glycosides, procyanidins, chlorogenic acid, anthocyanins
Grapes	Seed and skin	Cinnamic acid, coumaric acid, caffeic acid, ferulic acid, chlorogenic acid, neochlorogenic acid, p-hydroxybenzoic acid, protocatechuic acid, vanillic acid, gallic acid, proanthocyanidins, quercetin 3-O-glucuronide, quercetin, resveratrol, pullulan
Citrus	Peel	Hesperidin, naringin, eriocitrin, narirutin
Banana	Peel	Gallocatechin, anthocyanins, delphinidin, cyaniding, catecholamine
Litchi	Pericarp, seeds	Cyanidin-3-glucosides, cyanidin-3-rutonoside, malvidin-3-glucoside gallic acid, epicatechin-3-gallate
Mango	Kernel	Gallic acid, ellagic acid, gallates, gallotannins, condensed tannins

Source: Varzakas *et al.*, 2016

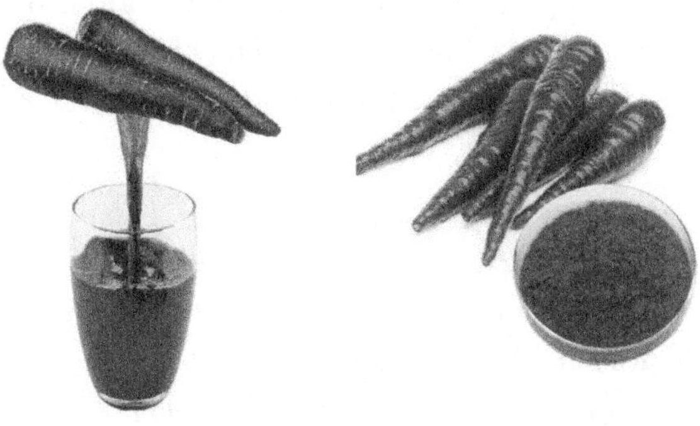

Fig. 15. Black carrot

Moreover, the phenolic portion of the peel shows L-tryptophane, p-coumaric and ferulic acids, as well as cyclo-DOPA glucoside derivatives. Beets are ranked among the ten most potent vegetables for antioxidant capacity, with a total phenolic content of 50–60 mmol/g dry weight (Schieber *et al.,* 2001). Besides that, lycopene is the principal carotenoid, which is responsible for the redness in tomatoes. The skin of a tomato is a rich source of lycopene, which is an essential component of waste originating from tomato paste manufacturing units. Several epidemiological studies have found that lycopene-rich diets are beneficial for human health. So, tomatoes and tomato products may lead to the prevention of cardiovascular disease and protection against certain types of cancer (Kosseva, 2013).

2. PROCESSING OF VEGETABLES FOR RECOVERY OF HIGH-VALUE PRODUCTS

1. Potato Peel Waste

In general, the losses caused by potato peeling range from 15% to 40%, depending upon the process exploited, i.e., steam, abrasion or lye peeling (Schieber *et al.,* 2001). PPW contains sufficient amounts of starch, cellulose, hemicellulose and fermentable sugars and hence used as an ethanol feedstock. The potato processing industries generate a large amount of starchy wastewater which should be treated before directed to the landfill as it may cause serious environmental problems due to high chemical oxygen demand (COD), biological oxygen demand (BOD) and suspended solids (SS).

Moreover, a study by (Muniraj *et al.,* 2015) investigated the bioconversion of potato processing wastewater into lipid-rich biomass using two oleaginous fungi- *Aspergillus flavus* I16-3 and *Mucor rouxii.* This study demonstrated an alternative approach to vaporise potato-processing wastewater to produce microbial lipids and g-linolenic acid (GLA) nutraceuticals.

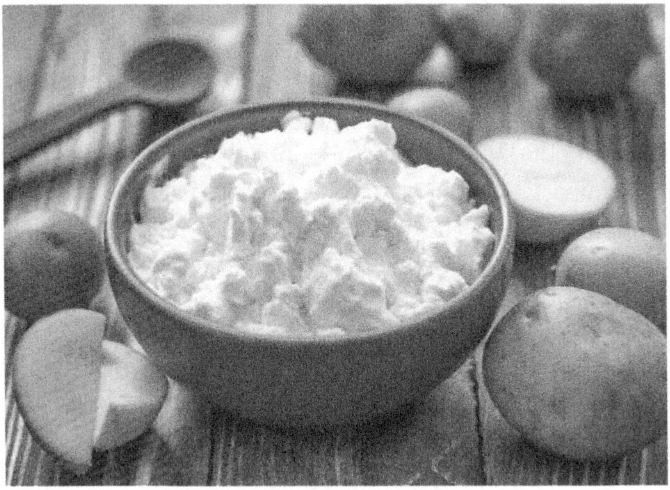

Fig. 16. Potato starch

2. Pistachio Hulls

Pistachio hulls are the promising source of primary (mainly protein and fat) and secondary (mainly phenol derivatives) metabolites. Further, they are also rich in minerals, vitamins and essential oils as found by Chahed *et al.* (2007) and Goli *et al.* (2005). Besides, Rajaei *et al.* (2010) analysed its anti-microbial and antimutagenicity activities and Barreca *et al.* (2016) extracted the hulls of ripe pistachios using two organic solvents (ethanol and methanol) and distinguished them for phenolic content, antioxidant capacity and cytoprotective activity.

3. Pumpkin

The seeds of pumpkins (*Cucurbita* sp.) are promising sources of lipid, protein, and ash. Further, they are also rich in mono and polyunsaturated fatty acids and have low levels of sugars, starches (Applequist *et al.*, 2006). The non-germinated seeds also contain antioxidants, anticancer, and anti-inflammatory properties (Adams *et al.,* 2011). Further, they also contain carotenoids, phenolic compounds, tocopherols and high amount of macronutrients.

4. Red Radish

The uses of anthocyanins are well known as natural colourants due to their colour characteristics along with the health benefits as antioxidants (Matsufuji *et al.*, 2007; Rahman *et al.*, 2006). Red radish (*Raphanus* L.) pickle is an important fermented vegetable product due to its colourful and textural properties. This kind of pickles are prepared in tons for consumption purpose, in this process, a considerable amount of radish brine is generated as a waste, which is a challenge for utilisation of radish brines rich in phytochemicals, colour properties, and antioxidant activities, produced during lactic acid fermentation. A study conducted by (Jing *et al.* 2014) on the phytochemicals and the antioxidative activities of red radish fermentation waste suggested further utilization of byproducts as nutraceuticals or natural colourants.

CHAPTER 11

NUTRACEUTICAL DELIVERY VEHICLES

In order to enhance the bioavailability of hydrophobic bioactive compounds in food, they are first isolated from their natural environments such as a fruit or vegetable and then incorporated into an appropriate delivery system (McClements *et al.*, 2010). A wide range of colloidal delivery systems are available to encapsulate bioactive agents, such as molecular complexes, microemulsions, emulsions, liposomes, stable lipid nanoparticles, biopolymer particles, and microgels. The utilisation of delivery approaches using a formulation with substances with a history of use in man has the potential to promote solubility, stability, or permeability of nutraceuticals, resulting in improved oral bioavailability. Major nutraceutical delivery vehicles are described below in details.

1. LIPOSOMES

Liposomes are spherical microscopic lipid vesicles shaped from phospholipids holding a little quantity of solvent within which they exist. They function as a delivery vehicle for both the hydrophilic and lipophilic compounds. Once the hydrophilic compounds are encapsulated, the aqueous centre of liposome serves as a suitable pocket for carrying the bioactive through the journey of the gastrointestinal (GI) tract digestion and absorption. Liposomes boost the oral bioavailability of a range of nutraceuticals, like curcumin and resveratrol, by entrapping them within the phospholipid bilayers (Takahashi *et al.,* 2009; El-Samaligy *et al.,*2006). The encapsulation raises the liquid solubility, protects against unstable stimuli, modulating intestinal absorption, and facilitating lymphatic transport.

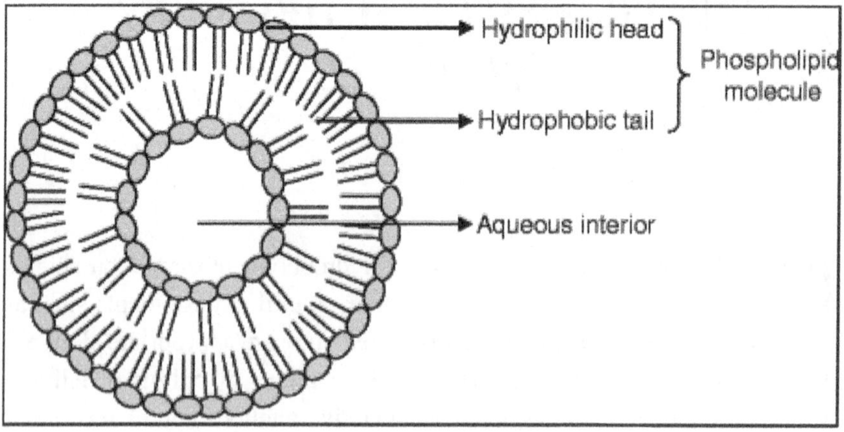

Fig. 17. Structure of a unilamellar liposome

2. PHOSPHOLIPID BASED

Phospholipids-based nanotherapeutics (Burgo *et al.,* 2014) gaining popularity currently as delivery vehicles as a result of their biocompatibility, biodegradable nature and possess properties that can enhance their bioavailability. When engaged in the aqueous environment, phospholipids at the same time adapt themselves into a bilayer structure.

3. NIOSOMES

The distinctive structures of niosomes are capable of encapsulating both hydrophilic and lipophilic substances. Tavano *et al.* (2014) reported that niosomes are delivery vehicles used for the encapsulation of antioxidants.

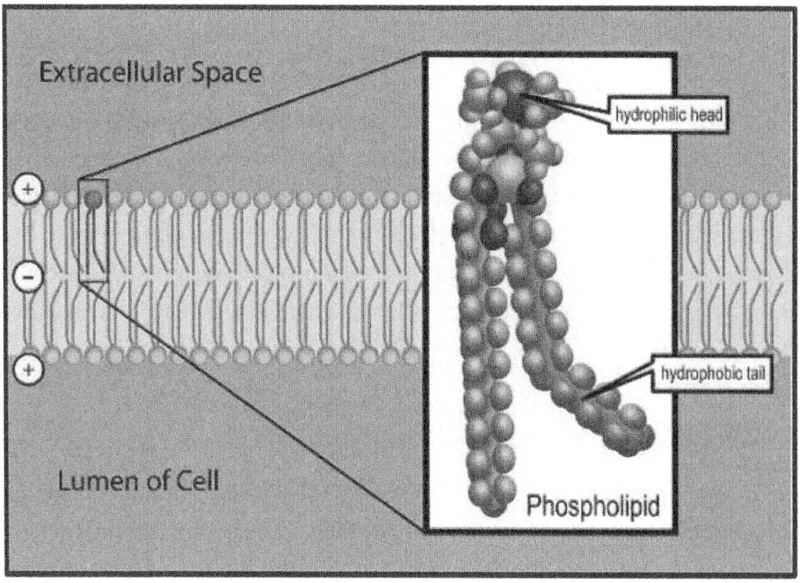

Fig. 18. Phospholipid structure

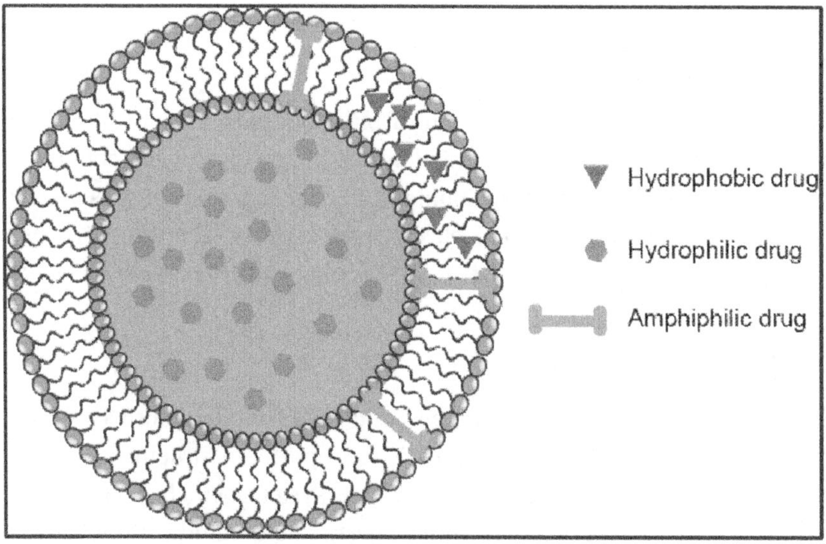

Fig. 19. Schematic representation of niosome

4. EMULSION-BASED DELIVERY VEHICLES

Because of their small particle size—usually >100 nm—and their ability to be formulated with generally recognised as safe (GRAS) material, emulsions are being employed extensively for the delivery of nutraceuticals. Nanoemulsion based oral formulations considerably enhance the absorption of nutraceuticals like curcumin, alpha-tocopherol when compared to their nonencapsulated forms. Emulsion based delivery systems enhance the solubility of different nutraceuticals such as quercetin, curcumin, resveratrol, Vitamin D3 (Ozturk *et al.*, 2015; Mukherjee *et al.*, 2015).

5. MICROEMULSIONS/NANOEMULSIONS

The droplet diameter of microemulsion (ME) is less than 100 nm, are spontaneous structures of water, oil, and surfactants. Microemulsions are employed to enhance the solubility of poorly water-soluble drugs or nutraceuticals in liquid solutions, either for the penetration or absorption by cells in the pharmaceutical and functional foods (Lin *et al.*, 2014).

6. ETHOSOMES

Ethosomes are primarily composed of phospholipids, ethanol (relatively high concentration, 40%–45%) and water, relatively higher content of ethanol makes efficient permeation and they are customarily inserted to vesicular systems to configure elastic nanovesicles. The dimensions of ethosomes vary between 30 nm to a few microns. (Shena *et al.*, 2014).

7. NANOENCAPSULATION

Submicron emulsion, also known as Solid-lipid nanoparticles (SLNs) are composed mainly of a solid or semisolid lipid core structure which is regarded as an excellent controlled-release system, which is capable of avoiding spurt release. They extend the gastric holding time of bioactives. SLNs have a robust protective mechanism against GI tract degradation activities (Yoo *et al.*, 2013; Maswal *et al.*,2013). Moreover, a delivery protein-mediated nanocarrier system exists there for hydrophobic nutraceuticals (especially those derived from milk) that represent a well-tolerated system with few side effects (Kimpel *et al.*, 2015).

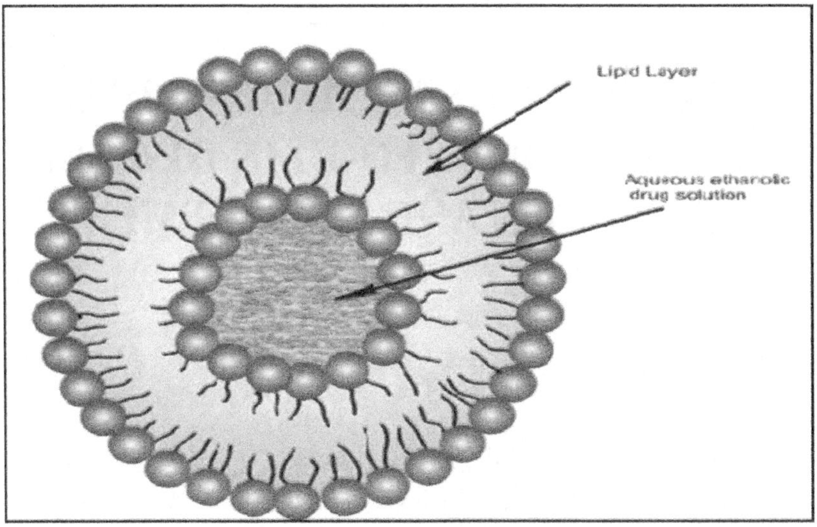

Fig. 20. Ethosome structure

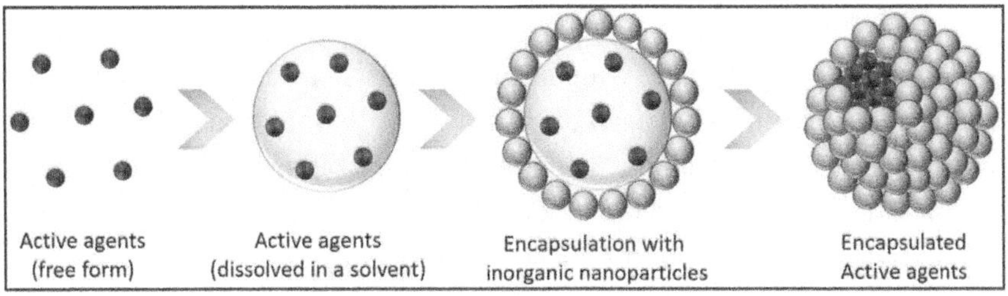

Fig. 21. Nanoencapsulation process

CHAPTER 12

ADVANTAGES OF NUTRACEUTICALS OR FUNCTIONAL FOOD IN DISEASE PREVENTION AND MANAGEMENT

1. It avoids side effect.
2. It may enhance the health beneficial effect.
3. It may have naturally dietary supplement; therefore, they do not have unpleasant side effects.
4. It may promote the health value, our diet and improves the medical condition of human.
5. Disease management with nutraceuticals derived from plant food residues: Fruit and vegetable wastes (FVW) are generated in large quantities in the markets, which constitute a big problem in municipal landfills due to their rapid biodegradability. Such residues are of great importance because of the phenolic compounds embedded within them, which impart nutraceutical properties to fruit residues. The natural, as well as synthetic antioxidants, are reported to have biological properties, such as anticarcinogenic, antimutagenic, antiallergenic, and antiaging.
6. It may easily be available and economically affordable (Chauhan *et al.*, 2013)

CHAPTER 13

CONCLUSION

With the change of time, human food habits are changing. Some are shifting toward the positive side and these people have a better knowledge about the maintenance of their balanced diet and proper nutrition, leading a good healthy life with overall fitness. In contrast, some people adopt unhealthy food habits. They tend to consume junk foods, smoke cigarettes and consume alcohol. This food behaviour ultimately leads to a condition, where antioxidant defence systems are often overloaded, resulting in oxidative stress due to excess free radicles and less antioxidant scavengers. It may result in uncountable problems like ageing, early wrinkles on the face, constipation, formation of melanin, acidity, gastric problems. Oxidative stress may further exacerbate various devastating diseases like cancer, heart-related problems, liver inflammation, weak immune and nervous system disorders. These factors altogether contribute towards a decreased life of a human with increased vulnerability to diseases leading an unhealthy life.

So, the wise option to prevent this oxidative damage is nutraceuticals. Consumption of fruits and vegetables rich in nutraceuticals (antioxidants) such as apple and strawberry, with full of phytochemicals in the form of anthocyanins, carotenoids, xanthophylls and ascorbic acid will be the solution as they engulf the reactive species of free radicals preventing oxidation leading to reduced oxidative stress. However, regular consumption of fruits and vegetables may not be feasible for everyone. Here the concept of Functional foods arises, which may be economical when prepared by using plant food residues as a source of nutraceutical. So, special attention should be given on the extraction of bioactive compounds from inexpensive or residual sources making nutraceutical available to every individual. It requires the tremendous efforts from the side of health professionals, nutritionists, biotechnologists, regulatory toxicologist and nutraceutical industrialist they must strategically work together to prepare a plan of work and appropriate regulation to provide the ultimate health and therapeutic benefits to humankind with purity, efficacy, and safety. Nutraceuticals have proven health benefits and their consumption (within their acceptable Recommended Dietary Intakes) will keep diseases at bay and allow humans to maintain an overall good health (Das *et al.*, 2012). The nutraceuticals present in the fruits and vegetables, if harnessed effectively, will uplift the economic significance of the fruits and vegetables. As the market demand of nutraceuticals is ever-growing, so there is an urgent need to explore the potentiality of fruits and vegetables in the field of nutraceuticals.

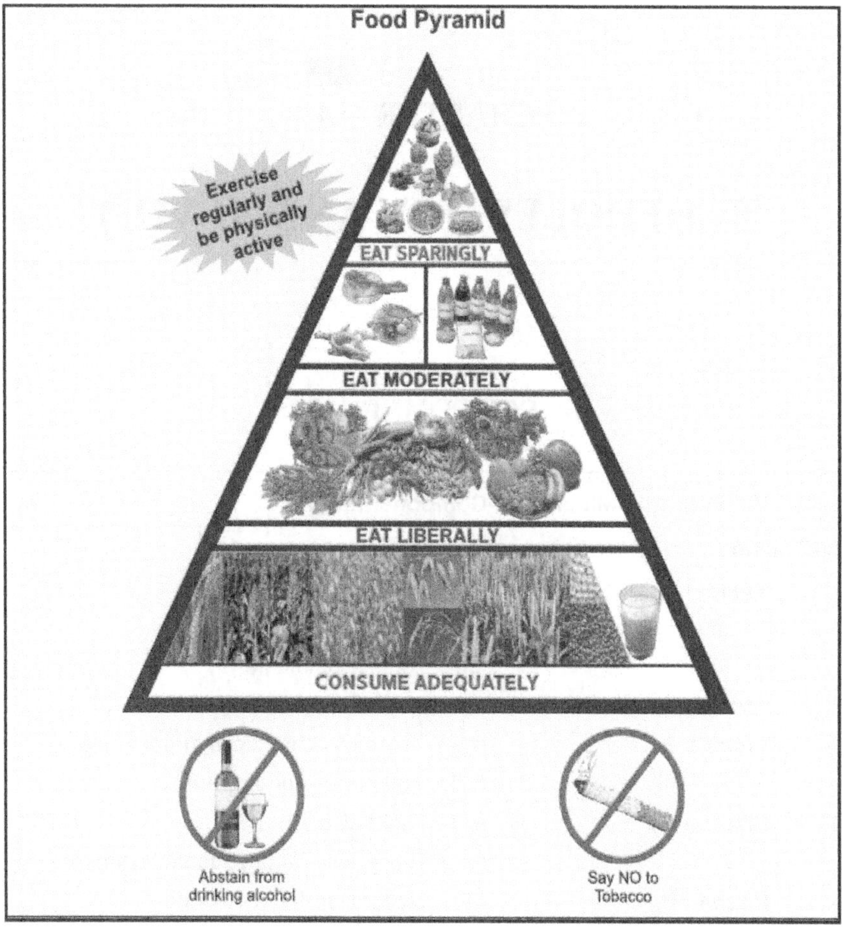

Fig. 22. Food pyramid

Source: FAO

CHAPTER 14

SCHEDULES (I-IV AND VI-VIII)

SCHEDULE – I

S.No.	Vitamins and Minerals	Components	
A. Vitamins			
1.	Vitamin A	(i)	Retinol - all trans retinol
		(ii)	Retinyl acetate
		(iii)	Retinyl palmitate
2.	Provitamin A	(i)	Beta-Carotene
3.	Vitamin B_1	(i)	Thiamine chloride hydrochloride
		(ii)	Thiamine mononitrate
4.	Vitamin B_2	(i)	Riboflavin
		(ii)	Riboflavin 5'- phosphate, sodium
5.	Vitamin B_6	(i)	Pyridoxine hydrochloride
		(ii)	Pyridoxal 5'-phosphate
6.	Vitamin B_{12}	(i)	Cyanocobalamin
		(ii)	Hydroxocobalamin
7.	Vitamin C	(i)	L-ascorbic acid
		(ii)	Sodium-L-ascorbate
		(iii)	Calcium-L-ascorbate

[Table Contd.

Contd. Table]

S.No.	Vitamins and Minerals	Components	
		(iv)	Potassium-L-ascorbate
		(v)	6-palmitoyl-L-ascorbic acid
		(vi)	Ascorbyl palmitate
8.	**Vitamin D**	(i)	Vitamin D3 (cholecalciferol) - Animal source
		(ii)	Vitamin D2 (ergocalciferol) - Plant source
9.	**Vitamin E**	(i)	D-alpha-tocopherol
		(ii)	DL-alpha-tocopherol
		(iii)	D-alpha-tocopheryl acetate
		(iv)	DL-alpha-tocopheryl acetate
		(v)	D-alpha-tocopheryl acid succinate
		(vi)	DL-alpha-tocopheryl acid succinate
		(vii)	DL-alpha-tocopheryl polyethylene glycol succinate
10.	**Vitamin K_1**	(i)	Phylloquinone
		(ii)	Phytomenadione (2-methyl 3-phytyl-1)
		(iii)	1,4-napthoquinone
		(iv)	Phytonamidione
11.	**Vitamin K_2 (MK-7)**	(i)	Menaquinone
12.	**Vitamin K_2 (MK-4)**	(i)	Menatetrenone
13.	**Biotin**	(i)	D-biotin
14.	**Folic Acid**	(i)	n-pteroyl-l-glutamic acid
15.	**Niacin**	(i)	Nicotinic acid
		(ii)	Nicotinamide
		(iii)	Nicotinic acid amide
16.	**Pantothenic acid**	(i)	D-pantothenate, calcium
		(ii)	D-pantothenate, sodium
		(iii)	D-panthenol
		(iv)	DL- panthenol
		(v)	Sodium-D-pantothenate

[Table Contd.

Note. Addition of appropriate overages to ensure adequate availability of vitamins in the products shall be permitted based on scientific rationale. However, the maximum proportion of overages shall not exceed as given in the Table 'C', below, unless scientifically justified. Labels of such products shall make a declaration of the same as "appropriate overages added" in the composition declaration Panel.

B. Minerals (Chemical sources)

S.No.	Vitamins and Minerals	Components
1.	Calcium	(i) Calcium carbonate
		(ii) Calcium chloride
		(iii) Calcium salts of citric acid
		(iv) Calcium gluconate
		(v) Calcium glycerophosphate
		(vi) Calcium orthophosphate
		(vii) Calcium hydroxide
		(viii) Calcium oxide
		(ix) Calcium phosphate, monobasic
		(x) Calcium phosphate, dibasic
		(xi) Calcium phosphate, tribasic
		(xii) Calcium sulphate
		(xiii) Calcium from algal source (Algus calcarius)
		(xiv) Calcium lactate
2.	Chloride	(i) Calcium chloride
		(ii) Choline chloride
		(iii) Magnesium chloride
		(iv) Manganese chloride
		(v) Potassium chloride
		(vi) Sodium chloride
3.	Chromium	(i) Chromium (III) chloride
		(ii) Chromium (III) sulphate

[Table Contd.

Contd. Table]

S.No.	Vitamins and Minerals	Components
4.	**Copper**	(i) Cupric carbonate
		(ii) Cupric citrate
		(iii) Cupric gluconate
		(iv) Cupric sulphate
		(v) Copper lysine complex
5.	**Iodine**	(i) Sodium iodide
		(ii) Sodium iodate
		(iii) Potassium iodide
		(iv) Potassium iodate
6.	**Iron**	(i) Ferrous succinate
		(ii) Ferrous citrate
		(iii) Ferric ammonium citrate
		(iv) Ferrous gluconate
		(v) Ferrous fumarate
		(vi) Ferric sodium di-phosphate
		(vii) Ferrous lactate
		(viii) Ferrous sulphate
		(ix) Ferric di-phosphate
		(x) Ferric saccharate
		(xi) Ferrous bis-glycinate
		(xii) Hydrogen reduced iron
		(xiii) Sodium Iron EDTA
		(xiv) Carbonyl iron
		(xv) Ferrous orthophosphate
		(xvi) Ferrous sodium pyrophosphate
		(xvii) Elemental iron
		(xviii) Electrolytic iron

[Table Contd.

Contd. Table]

S.No.	Vitamins and Minerals	Components
7.	**Magnesium**	(i) Magnesium aspartate
		(ii) Magnesium carbonate
		(iii) Magnesium chloride
		(iv) Magnesium gluconate
		(v) Magnesium phosphate dibasic (Magnesium hydrogen phosphate)
		(vi) Magnesium phosphate tribasic (Trimagnesium phosphate)
		(vii) Magnesium oxide
		(viii) Magnesium sulphate
8.	**Manganese**	(i) Manganese carbonate
		(ii) Manganese chloride
		(iii) Manganese citrate
		(iv) Manganese sulphate
		(v) Manganese gluconate
		(vi) As amino acid chelate
9.	**Molybdenum**	(i) Ammonium molybdate (Molybdenum (VI)
		(ii) Sodium molybdate (Molybdenum (VI)
		(iii) As amino acid chelate
10.	**Phosphorous**	(i) Potassium glycerophosphate
		(ii) Potassium phosphate, monobasic
		(iii) Potassium phosphate, dibasic
11.	**Potassium**	(i) Potassium bicarbonate
		(ii) Potassium carbonate
		(iii) Potassium chloride
		(iv) Potassium citrate
		(v) Potassium gluconate
		(vi) Potassium glycerophosphate
		(vii) Potassium lactate

[Table Contd.

Contd. Table]

S.No.	Vitamins and Minerals	Components	
		(viii)	Potassium monobasic phosphate
		(ix)	Potassium dibasic phosphate
12.	**Selenium**	(i)	Sodium selenate
		(ii)	Sodium selenite
		(iii)	Sodium hydrogen selenite
		(iv)	Selenomethionine
13.	**Sodium**	(i)	Sodium bicarbonate
		(ii)	Sodium carbonate
		(iii)	Sodium chloride
		(iv)	Sodium citrate (Trisodium citrate)
		(v)	Sodium gluconate
		(vi)	Sodium lactate
		(vii)	Sodium phosphate monobasic (Sodium dihydrogen phosphate)
		(viii)	Sodium phosphate dibasic (disodium hydrogen phosphate)
		(ix)	Sodium sulphate
14.	**Zinc**	(i)	Zinc acetate
		(ii)	Zinc chloride
		(iii)	Zinc citrate
		(iv)	Zinc gluconate
		(v)	Zinc lactate
		(vi)	Zinc oxide
		(vii)	Zinc carbonate
		(viii)	Zinc sulphate
15.	**Boron**	(i)	Boron proteonate

Note. Suitable esters and salts of vitamins and salts and chelates of minerals may be used.

[Table Contd.

Contd. Table]

C. Permissible overages*

S.No.	Micronutrient	Overage (per cent)
1.	Vitamin A	30
2.	Vitamin C	20
3.	Vitamin D	30
4.	Vitamin E	10
5.	Thiamine (vitamin B_1)	25
6.	Riboflavin (vitamin B_2)	25
7.	Niacin (vitamin B_3)	10
8.	Vitamin B_6	25
9.	Vitamin B_{12}	25
10.	Folic acid	25
11.	Pantothenic acid	10
12.	Vitamin K_1	30
13.	Minerals	10
14.	Iodine	20

Source: FSSAI

* Overage means the amount of excess nutrients added above label claim during manufacture as a means of maintaining at least the claimed amount of the ingredient(s) for the normal shelf life of the product to compensate for the expected manufacturing/storage loss and to allow for variation in assay performance. Where overages are more than those listed in **Schedule I, Table C,** the same shall be scientifically substantiated.

[Table Contd.

SCHEDULE – II

List of Amino Acids and Other Nutrients

A. Essential Amino Acids

(i) L-Histidine
(ii) L-Histidine hydrochloride
(iii) L-Isoleucine
(iv) L-Isoleucine hydrochloride
(v) L-Leucine
(vi) L-Leucine hydrochloride
(vii) L-Lysine
(viii) L-Lysine hydrochloride
(ix) DL-Methionine
(x) L-Cysteine
(xi) L-Cysteine hydrochloride
(xii) L-Aspartic acid
(xiii) L-Arginine L-aspartate
(xiv) L-Threonine
(xv) L- Alanine
(xvi) L-Phenylalanine
(xvii) L-Cysteine hydrochloride
(xviii) L-Tyrosine
(xix) L-Arginine
(xx) L-Tryptophan
(xxi) L-Valine
(xxii) L-Arginine hydrochloride

B. Non- Essential Amino Acids

(i) L-Carnitine
(ii) L-Carnitine hydrochloride
(iii) Carnitine, acetyl-L
(iv) L-Glutamic acid
(v) L-Glutamine
(vi) Glycine
(vii) L-Hydroxylysine
(viii) L-Hydroxyproline
(ix) L-Lycine acetate
(x) N-acetyl-L-cysteine
(xi) L- Ornithine
(xii) L-Ornithine monohydrochloride
(xiii) L-Lycine –L- aspartate
(xiv) L-Citruline
(xv) L- Proline
(xvi) L-Lycine-L-glutamate dihydrate
(xvii) Megnesium L- aspartate
(xviii) Calcium L- glutamate
(xix) Potassium – L- glutamate
(xx) Carnitine tartrate
(xxi) Taurine
(xxii) Choline
(xxiii) Choline chloride
(xxiv) Choline citrate
(xxv) L-Serine
(xxvi) Tyrosine, acetyl-L
(xxvii) Choline hydrogen tartrate
(xxviii) Myo-inositol

C. Nucleotides

(i) Adenosine 5-monophosphate (AMP)

(ii) Cystidine 5-mono phosphate (CMP)

(iii) Guanosine 5-mono phosphate (GMP)

(iv) Inosine 5-mono phosphate (IMP)

(v) Disodium uridine 5-monophosphate

(vi) Disodium guanosine 5-mono phosphate

(vii) Disodium ionosine 5-mono phosphate

Source: FSSAI

Note. Suitable esters and salts of amino acids may be used.

SCHEDULE - III

Values for vitamins, minerals and trace elements allowed to be used in food for special dietary use and food for special medical purpose (other than those intended for use ininfant formula)

1. Vitamins

Vitamins	RDA for Vitamins			
	Per 100 kJ		Per 100 kcal	
	Minimum	Maximum*	Minimum	Maximum*
Vitamin A (μg RE)	8.4	43	35	180
Vitamin D (μg)	0.12	0.65 (0.75)[1]	0.5 (3)[1]	2.5
Vitamin K (μg)	0.85	5	3.5	20
Vitamin C (mg)	0.54	5.25	2.25	22
Thiamin (mg)	0.015	0.12	0.06	0.5
Riboflavin (mg)	0.02	0.12	0.08	0.5
Vitamin B_6 (mg)	0.02	0.12	0.08	0.5
Niacin (mg NE)	0.22	0.75	0.9	3
Folic acid (μg)	2.5	12.5	10	50
Vitamin B_{12} (μg)	0.017	0.17	0.07	0.7
Pantothenic acid (mg)	0.035	0.35	0.15	1.5
Biotin (μg)	0.18	1.8	0.75	7.5
Vitamin E (mg α-TE)	0.5/g of polyunsaturated fatty Acids expressed as linoleic acid but in no case less than 0.1 mg per 100 available kJ	0.75	0.5/g of polyunsaturated fatty Acids expressed Aslinoleic acid but in no case less 0.1 mg per 100 available kcal	3

(1): For products intended for children of 1 to 10 years of age;

NE – Niacin equivalent;

TE – Tocopherol equivalent.* When no upper safe level (maximum permissible level higher than 1 (100 percent) RDA) has been specified for particular vitamins and minerals, the content of such nutrient shall not exceed NOAEL (No observed adverse effect level) or one-tenth of LOAEL (Lowest observed adverse effect level)

2. Minerals

Minerals	RDA for Minerals			
	Per 100kJ		Per 100 kcal	
	Minimum	Maximum*	Minimum	Maximum*
Sodium (mg)	7.2	42	30	175
Chloride (mg)	7.2	42	30	175
Potassium (mg)	19	70	80	295
Calcium (mg)	8.4	42	35	175
	(12)[1]	(60)[1]	(50)[1]	(250)[1]
Phosphorus (mg)	7.2	19	30	80
Magnesium (mg)	1.8	6	7.5	25
Iron (mg)	0.12	0.5	0.5	2.0
Zinc (mg)	0.12	0.36	0.5	1.5
Copper (µg)	15	125	60	500
Iodine (µg)	1.55	8.4	6.5	35
Selenium (µg)	0.6	2.5	2.5	10
Manganese (mg)	0.012	0.12	0.05	0.5
Chromium (µg)	0.3	3.6	1.25	15
Molybdenum (µg)	0.72	4.3	3.5	18

(1): For products intended for children of 1 to 10 years of age;*When no upper safe level (maximum permissible level higher that 1 (100 per cent) RDA) has been specified for a particular nutrient the content of such nutrient shall not exceed NOAEL (No observed adverse effect level) or one-tenthof LOAEL (Lowest observed adverse effect level)

Source: FSSAI

SCHEDULE – IV

List of plant or botanical ingredients

S.No.	Botanical name and part used	Official and common names	Permitted range of usage for adults per day (given in terms of raw herb/ material)
1.	*Abelmoschus esculentus* (L.) Moench.		
	Fruit/Root	Bhindi	5-10 g (as powder)
2.	*Abies spectabilis (D.Don) / A. pindrow* Royle / *Abies webbiana* Lindl (syn)		
	Leaf/ Fruit	Talis patra / Talis bhed	2-3 g (as powder)
3.	*Asculus indica colebr./ A. hippocastanum*		
	Fruit /Kernel Extract	Ban-khoda / Indian Horse Chestnut	3 – 5 g (as powder) 300 – 500 mg
4.	*Abelmoschus moschatus / Hibiscus abelmoschus* (syn)		
	Seed	*Lata kasturi*	1-2 g
5.	*Abutilon indicum* (L.) Sweet ssp. *indicum / A. fruiticosum*		
	Seed/Root / Stem	Atibala / kanghibala	3 – 4 g (as powder)
6.	*Acacia arabica* Willd. (Now known as *Acacia nilotica* (L.) Willd. ex Del. ssp. *indica* (Benth.) Brenan		
	Gum Bark	Babbul	1-3 g 5-10 g

7.	*Acacia catechu*		
	Extract / heartwood	Khadir/ Katha/khair	1-3 g
8.	*Acacia leucophloea* Willd/A. farnesiana (syn)		
	Bark/Leaf Seed/Gum	Airmed/Trimed	3-5 g 2-3 g
9.	*Achillea millefolium* Linn. / *A. Lanulosa* Nutt. (syn)		
	Leaf	Gandana/Biranjaasif	2-3 g (as powder)
10.	*Achyranthes aspera* (L.)/ *A. bidentala*		
	Seed/Plant	Apamarga / Chirchida	5-8 g (as powder)
11.	*Acorus calamus* Linn.		
	Leaf	Vachha/Waj/Vacha	60-125 mg (as powder)
12.	*Adhatoda zeylanica / A. vasaka*		
	Stem/ Leaf /Root/ Flower	Vasa / Adusa	5-10 g
13.	*Aegle marmelos* (L.) Corr.		
	Unripe fruit pulp	Bilwa / Bael	5-10 g (as pulp)
	Ripe fruit pulp		30-50 g (as pulp)
	Leaf/Bark	Bael Pather/ Bael chhal	3-6 g (as powder)
14.	*Ajuga bracteosa* Wall.		
	Plant	Neel Kanthi	0.5 – 1 g
15.	*Alangium salvifolium* (L.f.) Wang. ssp. *salvifolium / A. lamarckii* (syn)		
	Fruit	Ankota	2-6 g (as powder)

16.	*Albizia lebbeck* (L.) Benth/*A. procera*/*A. odoratissima*		
	Flower/ Stem bark / Leaf	Shireesh / Siris	3-6 g (as powder)
	Seed	Siris	1-3 g (as powder)
17.	*Alpinia galanga*		
	Rhizome	Kulanjan	1-3 g (as powder)
18.	*Allium cepa* L.		
	Bulb	Plandu / Pyaj	10-20 ml (as juice)
	Seed	Pyaj	1-3 g (as powder)
	Leaf		20-40 g (as fresh)
19.	*Allium sativum* L.		
	Bulb	Rason/ Lahsun	1-3 g (Not recommended during pregnancy)
	Leaf	Lahsun	10-20 g (as fresh)
20.	*Allium stracheyi* Bakerno		
	Whole plant	Farran	2-3 g
21.	*Alocasia indica* Spach (Now known as *A. macrorhiza* (L.) G. Don)		
	Tuber	Mankand / Kasnalu	5-10 g

22.	*Aloe barbadensis* Mill. / *A. Ferox* / *A. vera* / *A. indica*		
	Leaf	Kumari / Ghikvar / Ghrit kumari	5-10 g (as pulp)
	Dried Pulp	Elua -mussabar / kanyasar	0.5 – 1 g
23.	*Althaea officinalis* Linn.		
	Flower/Root	Khatmi / Resha-khatmi	3-6 g (as powder)
24.	*Alternanthera sessilis* (L.) R. Br. ex DC.		
	Whole plant	Matsyakshi / Gudarisaga	2-3 g (as powder)
25.	*Amaranthus gangeticus* L. (Now known as *A. tricolor* L.) / *A. blitum* L.		
	Aerial part	Maaraish / Lal marsa -sag / marsa	10-20 g (as fresh)
26.	*Amaranthus spinosus* L. / *A. paniculatus* L. (*A. hybridus* L.)		
	Whole plant	Tanduliya / Chaulai Kateli / Jal Chaulai	20-30 g (as fresh)
27.	*Amomum subulatum* Roxb./ A. aromaticum Roxb.		
	Fruit	Sthula- elaa / Badi Elaichi	1-3 g (as powder)
	Seed	Badi Elaichi	1-2 g (as powder)
28.	*Amorphophallus campanulatus* (Roxb.) Blume ex Decne.		
	Corm	Suran / Jimikand	20-50 g (as fresh)
29.	*Anacardium occidentale* L.		
	Fruit kernel	Kaju / Cashew nut	10-20 g

30.	*Anacyclus pyrethrum* DC.		
	Root/ Seed	Akarkar	100 - 250 mg (as powder) (Not recommended for children below 5 years)
31.	*Ananas comosus* (L.) Merr.		
	Fruit	Ananas / Pineapple	50-100 g (as fresh) 50-100 ml (as juice) (Not recommended during pregnancy)
32.	*Andrographis paniculata*		
	Whole plant	Kalmegh / Bhuunimba	1-3 g (as powder)
	Extract		125 - 250 mg
33.	*Anethum sowa* Roxb. ex Flem. (Now known as *A. graveolens* L.)		
	Fruit	Shataahvaa / Shatapushpa/ Sowa / Indian dill seed	3-6 g (as powder)
	Leaf	Sowa	10-20 g (as fresh)
34.	*Angelica glauca* Edgew./ *A. archangelica* L. / *A. himalaica* Krishna. & Badhwar.		
	Root / Root stock	Chandeo / Choraka / Chora	2-4 g (as powder)

35.	*Annona squamosa* L (Sitaphal)./*A. reticulata* (Ramphal)/*A. muricata* (Laxmanphal)/ *A. cherimola* (Hanuman phal)		
	Fruit pulp	Shareefa	20-30 g
	Leaf		3-5 g (as powder) (Not recommended for children below 16 years)
36.	*Apium leptophyllum* (Pers.) Muell. / *A. graveolens* Linn.		
	Fruit	Ajamod / Ajmoda bhed / celery	1-3 g (as powder)
37.	*Arachis hypogaea* L.		
	Seeds (kernel)	/ Mungphali / peanut / ground nut / sing dana	20-30 g
	Seed oil	Mungaphali tail	5-10 ml
38.	*Areca catechu* L.		
	Seed	Punga / Supari / Betel nut	1-2 g (as powder) (only to be used after shodhana (purification)) (Not recommended for children below 5 years)

39.	*Argyreia speciosa* Sweet / *A. nervosa* (syn)		
	Root	Vridharuka / Bridhara	3-5 g
	Seed		1-2 g
40.	*Armoracia lapathifolia* Gilib / *A .rusticana* Gaertn. (syn)		
	Leaf	Horse radish	2 -5 g
41.	*Artemisia absinthium* Linn / *A.vulgaris* / *A. officinalis* Linn / *A. maritima* / *A. dracunculus* / *A. annua*		
	Whole plant	Damanak / Afsantin / Chauhar /	1-2 g
42.	*Artocarpus heterophyllus* Lam. (Jackfruit)		
	Ripe / unripe fruit	Katahal	20-50 g
	Seeds		5-10 g
43.	*Artocarpus lakoocha* Roxb.		
	Ripe fruit / Unripe fruit	Lakuch / Badhal	20-30 g
	Seed	Badhal / Dhehu	5-10 g
44.	*Arnebia nobilis/A. benthamii*		
	Root	Ratanjot	2-4 g
45.	*Asparagus adscendens* Roxb.		
	Tuberous root	Musali / Safed musali	3-6 g (as powder)

46.	*Asparagus officinalis* L.		
	Root	Shatavari bhed	3-6 g (as powder)
	Tender Shoots		20-50 g
47.	*Asparagus racemosus* Willd.		
	Tuberous root	Shatawar	3-6 g (as powder)
	Tender Shoots		20-50 g
48.	*Asparagus sarmentosus* Linn.		
	Tuberous root	Badi shatawar	3-6 g (as powder)
49.	*Astragalus gummifer* Labill.		
	Gum	Kateeva gond (gum)/ Tragacanth gum	3-5 g
50.	*Avena sativa* L.		
	Seed	Oat	10-30 g (as powder)
51.	*Averrhoa carambola* L.		
	Fruit	Karmarang / Kamarakh	10-20 g

52.	*Azadirachta indica* A. Juss.		
	Leaf	Nimba / Neem / Margosa tree	1-3 g (as powder) (Not recommended for males and Females planning to conceive)
	Fruit	Neem	1-2 g (as pulp) (Not recommended for males and females planning to conceive) (Not recommended for children below 5 years)
	Flower		2-4 g (as powder)
	Bark / Root bark		3-6 g (as powder)
53.	*Bambusa arundinacea* (Retz.) Willd. / *B. bambos* Linn. (syn)		
	Tender shoots (Young leaf)	Bansh	20-30 g (as fresh)
	Seed	Bansh chaval	20-30 g (as powder)
	Crystals	Bansalochan	0.5-2 g (as powder)
54.	*Bacopa monnieri*		
	Whole plant	Brahmi	5-10 g (as fresh)
	Extract	Brahmi ghan	0.5 – 1 g

55.	*Basella alba* L.		
	Leaf	Poyi saag	20-30 g (as fresh)
56.	*Bauhinia variegata* L. / *B. purpurea*L. / *B. tomentosa*. Linn / *B. racemosa* / *B. malabarica*. Roxb.		
	Bark	Kachnar	1-3 g
	Flower / Buds	Kachnar / Kurvindar / Kovindar	10-20 ml (as juice)
	Extract		0.5 – 1 g
57.	*Benincasa hispida* (Thunb.) Cogn.		
	Fruit Seed	Kushmanda / Petha / Bhatua	30-50 g (as fresh) 5-10 g
58.	*Berberis aristata* DC./*B. asiatica* / *B. lycium* / *B. vulgaris*		
	Fruit / Leaf / Root / Stem	Daruhaldi / kashmall	5-10 g
	Root extract/ Stem extract	Rasaunt	0.5-1 g
59.	*Bergenia linguts* Wall / *B.ciliata*syn. / *Saxifraga lingulata* Wall.		
	Root/ Leaf	Pashanbhed / Pathar Chatta	10-20 g (for decoction) 3-6 g (as powder)

60.	*Beta vulgaris* L.		
	Tuber	Palanki / Chukandar	10-20 ml (as juice)
61.	*Blepharis edulis* Pers. / *B. linariaefolis*		
	Root Seed	Uttangan/ Karmavridhi	5-10 g (for decoction) 3-6 g
62.	*Boerhavia diffusa* L. (Now known as *B. repens* L. var. *diffusa* (L.) Hook.f.) / *B. Verticillata*		
	Aerial part	Punarnava / Itsit	20-30 g (for decoction) 1-3 g (as powder)
	Root	Bishkhapra	10-15 g (for decoction) 1-3 g (as powder)
63.	*Bombax malabarica / Salmalia malabarica / B. ceiba* L.		
	Bark	Shalmali / Semal / Semal Musali	5-10 g
	Flower		10-20 ml (as juice) 2-5 g (as powder)
	Gum/Root		1-3 g (as powder)
64.	*Boswellia serrata* Roxb.		
	Oleoresin	Shallaki / Kunduru / Salai guggal	1-3 g

65.	*Borassus flabellifer* L.		
	Dried inflorescence	Tarkul/Taad / Taadi	1-3 g (as powder)
	Seed pulp of unripe fruit		10-30 g
	Exudate of stem / sap		100-200 ml (as juice)
66.	*Brassica campestris* L. (Now known as *B. rapa* L. ssp. *campestris* (L.) Clapham)		
	Seed	Sarshap/ Sarson	10-20 g (as paste)
	Seed oil		10-20 ml
	Leaf		10-30 g (as fresh)
67.	*Brassica juncea* (L.) Czern./*B. nigra* Linn.		
	Seed	Rajikaa / Rai / Raai	1-2 g
	Leaf	Rai	10-20 g (as fresh)
68.	*Brassica rapa* L.		
	Tuber	Shalgam / Shaljam	20-40 g
	Leaf		20-30 g (as fresh)
69.	*Buchanania lanzan* Spreng.		
	Seed	Priyala / Chirounji	5-10 g (as powder)

70.	*Butea monosperma Taub / B. frondosa*		
	Seed	Palash / Dhark	1 – 3 g
	Gum Root/Bark		0.5-1.5 g 5-10 g (for decoction)
71.	*Bixa orellana* Linn.		
	Seed	Sindhuri / Annato Plant	1-3 g
72.	*Caesalpinia bonducella* (L.) Flem. (Now known as *C. bonduc* (L.) Roxb. *C.crista*)		
	Leaf /Bark / Seed	Putikaranj / Karanjuva / Latakaranja	2-3 g
73.	*Cajanus cajan* (Linn.) Millsp.		
	Seed	Adaki / Arahar / Tuvar ki daal	20-30 g
74.	*Camellia sinensis*		
	Tea leaf Extract	Chai patti Tea extract	Upto 10 g per day dried or processed leaf as infusion 1 – 2 g
	Tea catachins	Green tea catechins	0.3-1 g

75.	*Canavalia ensiformis* sensu Baker (Now known as *C. gladiata* (Jacq.) DC.)		
	Fresh pod Seed	Sem	30-50 g 5-10 g
76.	*Canscora decussata* (Roxb.) J.F. and J.H. Schult.		
	Leaf	Bangiya / Sankhapusphi	2-4 g (as powder)
77.	*Capparis decidua* (Forssk.) Edgew./ *C. aphylla* Edgew (syn)		
	Fruit	Kareer / Dela	10-20 g
78.	*Capparis seppiara* Linn. / *C. spinosa* Linn.		
	Root / Plant	Himsraa/ Kakadaani	5 – 10 g (as powder / for decoction)
79.	*Capsicum annum* L. var. *annum*		
	Unripe fruit	Hari Mirch	1-5 g (Not recommended for children below 5 years)
	Ripe fruit	Lal Mirch	0.5-1 g (as powder) (Not recommended for children below 5 years)
80.	*Capsicum frutescens* L.		
	Fruit	Simla mirch	30-50 g (as fresh)

81.	*Carica papaya* L.		
	Ripe fruit	Erand karkaki / Papita	50-100 g
	Unripe fruit	Papita	30 -50 g (Not recommended during pregnancy)
	Leaf/Juice	Papita	5 – 10 g/ml (for decoction) (Not recommended during pregnancy)
82.	*Carissa carandas* L. / *C. spinarum* L.		
	Fruit	Karmard / Karounda	10 – 20 g
	Bark	Garnaa	10-20 g (for decoction)
83.	*Carthamus tinctorius* L.		
	Flower / Leaf / Seed	Kusumbh / Barre	2-4 g (as powder)
	Seed oil	Barre –tail	5-10 ml
84.	*Carum carvi* L.		
	Fruit	Krishna jeerak/ Syaha /kala jeera	1-3 g (as powder)
85.	*Cassia absus* L.		
	Seed	Chakshushya / Chaksu	2-5 g

86.	*Cassia occidentalis* L.		
	Leaf	Kasmard / Kasoundi	5-10 g
	Seed / Fruit		1-3 g
87.	*Cassia tora* L. / *C. alata* L.		
	Leaf/Juice	Chakarmard / Chakwad	10-20 g/ml
	Seed		3-5 g (as powder)
88.	*Cassia fistula Linn.*		
	Fruit / Tender fruit	Aaragavadh / Amaltas	10-20 g (as pulp)
	Seed / Bark	Amaltas	2-5 g (as powder)
89.	*Cassia angustifolia/ C. acutifolia / C. senna* L		
	Seed/Leaf Extract	Swarnapatri / Sanay / Senna	0.5 – 2 g (as powder) 125 – 250 mg
90.	*Cedrus deodar* Roxb.		
	Seed/Wood/Bark Oil	Devdaru / Devdar	3-6 g (as powder) 2-4 ml
91.	*Celosia argentea* L. var. *argentea*		
	Seed	Shitivaaraka / Surwali / Safed murga	3-6 g

92.	*Celastrus paniculatus*		
	Seed Oil	Jyothishmati / Malkanguni	2 – 3 g (as powder) 1-2 ml
93.	*Celastrus paniculata* willd.		
	Seed Seed oil Leaf	Jyothishmati / Maalkangni	3-5g 5 - 15 drops 3-5 g (as powder)
94.	*Centella asiatica* (L.) Urban		
	Whole Plant Leaf	Mandukaparni / Brahmi (Galpatri) / Manduki	20-30 g (as fresh) 3-5 g (as powder)
	Extract	Brahmi	0.5 – 1 g
95.	*Centratherum anthelminticum*		
	Fruit/Seed	Aranya jeerak/ Kali-jeeri / Van-jeeri	1 – 3 g
96.	*Chenopodium album* L.		
	Whole plant/Leaf	Vasthuka/ Bathua	20-30 g (as fresh)
	Seed	Bathua	2-5 g
97.	*Chlorophytum borivillianum / C. arundinaceum/ C. tuberosum*		
	Root	Musali safed / Musali	3 – 6 g (as powder)
98.	*Cicca acida* (L.) Merrill		

98.	*Cicca acida* (L.) Merrill		
	Fruit	Harfa rewadi	10-20 g
99.	*Cicer arietinum* L.		
	Tender leaf	Chanak / Chana / Kalachana	30-50 g (as fresh)
	Seed	Chana / Kalachana	20-30 g
100.	*Cichorium endivia*		
	Seed/Root	Kasani/Chicory	5-10 g
101.	*Cinnamomum tamala* Nees/ Eberm. / *C. wightii*		
	Leaf	Tamalpatra/ Tejapatra	2-3 g
102.	*Cinnamomum zeylanicum* Blume (Now known as *C. verum* J. S. Presl.)/ *C. cassia* (syn) / *C. aromaticum*		
	Bark	Twak / Dalchini (Ceyloni)	1-2 g (Not recommended during pregnancy)
103.	*Cissampelos pareria* L. var. *hirsuta* (Buch. Ham. ex DC.) Forman.		
	Leaf / Whole Plant/ Root	Patha/ Padhi	3 – 6 g (as powder)
104.	*Cissus quadrangularis* L.		
	Aerial part	Astisamhara / Hadjod	20-30 g (as fresh)
	Stem	Hadjod	3-6 g
	Extract		0.5 – 1 g

105.	*Citrullus colocynthis* (L.) Schard.		
	Fruit / Root / Leaf	Indarvaruni / Indarun / Indrayan	0.25-0.5 g (as powder) (Not recommended during pregnancy)
106.	*Citrullus vulgaris* Schrad. ex Eckl.and Zeyh. var. *fistulosus* (Stocks) Stewart		
	Fruit	Tinda	20-40 g (as fresh)
107.	*Citrullus lanatus* (Thunb.) Matsura and Nakai		
	Fruit	Tarbuj	50-100 g (as pulp)
	Seed		3-6 g
	Seed oil		1-3 ml
108.	*Citrus aurantifolia* (Christm. and Panz.) Swingle / *C. medica* / *C. acida*. Roxb.		
	Fruit / Leaf / Root	Nimbuca / Nimbu	3-5 ml (as juice)
109.	*Citrus limon* (Linn.) Burm.f.		
	Fruit / Leaf / Root	Jambeer / Jameerinibu	5-10 ml (as juice)
110.	*Citrus maxima* (Burm.)Merr./ *C.grandis* L		
	Fruit / Leaf	Chakotara / Sadaphala	30-50 g (as fresh) 5-10 ml (as juice)
111.	*Citrus medica* L.var.medica		
	Fruit	Turanuj / Bijoura	5-10 ml (as juice)

112.	*Citrus reticulata* Blanc.		
	Fruit / Leaf	Narangi / Santra	30-50 ml (as juice)
113.	*Citrus sinensis* (L.) Osbeck		
	Fruit / Leaf	Mousami	50-100 ml (as juice)
114.	*Clerodendron infortunatum*		
	Whole plant	Bhandiri / Bhaandi / Bhatechh	10 – 20 ml (as juice)
115.	*Clerodendrum phlomidis*		
	Whole plant	Arani / Laghuagnimandh	10-20 g (for decoction) 3-5 g (as powder)
115.	*Clerodendrum serratum*		
	Whole plant	Bharangi	3-6 g (as powder)
116.	*Clitoria ternatea* Linn.		
	Root/Seed Leaf	Girikarnika / Aparajita	1-3 g 2-5 g (as powder)
117.	*Coccinia grandis* (L.) Voigt. / *C. indica* / *C. cardifolia* (syn)		
	Leaf	Bimbi/ Kundru phal / Kuntru shak	5-10 g (Not recommended for children below 5 years)

	Stem	Kundru	3-6 g (as powder)
	Whole plant	Kundru	3-6 g (as powder) 5-10 ml (as juice)
	Fruit	Kundru	20-50 g (as fresh)
118.	*Cocos nucifera* L.		
	Endosperm	Nariyal	10-20 g
	Water	Nariyal jala	100-200 ml
	Flower	Nariyal	5-10 g
	Shell / Fibre / Whole fruit	Ash	125 – 250 mg
119.	*Cocculus hirsutus* (L.) Theob.		
	Leaf / Whole plant	Chilihintha / Jalajamani	10-20 g (for decoction) 2 – 4 g (as powder)
120.	*Coix lacryma-jobi* L.		
	Seed	Millet/ Gavedhukaa/ Gargari	10-20 g
121.	*Coffea arabica / C. robusta*		
	Seed (Dry/Green)	Kaaphi / Kahava / Coffee	3-5 g (Not recommended for children below 5 years)

122.	*Coleus forskohlii / C. aromaticus / C. barbatus* (syn)		
	Root / Leaf / Whole plant	Gandiva / Pathachoor / Parn-yavani	3-5 g (as powder) (Not recommended for children below 5 years)
123.	*Coleus vettiveroides* K.C. Jacob.		
	Stem / Leaf / Root	Hrivera / Baalatka	3-5 g (as powder)
124.	*Coleticum luteum* Baker		
	Corm	Suranjan / Suranjan-kadvi	0.5 - 1 g (Not recommended in children below 5 years and pregnant mothers)
125.	*Colocasia antiquorum* Schott. (Now known as *C. esculenta* (L.) Schott.)		
	Rhizome	Pindalaka/ Arvi/ Aaluki	20-30 g (as fresh) (Not recommended for children below 16 years)
126.	*Commelina bengalensis* L.		
	Whole plant	Karnsphota / karnmorata / Kausar	3-6 g

127.	*Commiphora wightii*		
	Oleoresin	Guggal	2-4 g (Not recommended
			for children below 5 years)
128.	*Commiphora myrrha*		
	Oleoresin	Hirabol	2-4 g (Not recommended for children below 5 years)
129.	*Convolvulus pluricaulis / Evolvus alsinoides*		
	Whole plant (with white or bluish flowers)	Shankh-pushpi / Vishnukranta	10-20 g (for decoction)
130.	*Convolvulus turpethum I Iporius turpethum*		
	Root / Seed	Sygma-kali nishoth / Safed Nishoth	2-4 g (as powder)
131.	*Coptis teeta* Wall. / *C. chinensis* syn		
	Whole plant	Mamira / Tiktamoola	1-3 g (as powder)
132.	*Corchorus acutangulus* Lam. (Now known as *C. aestuans* L.) / *C. capasularis L / C. olitorius* L		
	Aerial part	Chunchu / kaala / shaak / palva saag / Chench	10-20 ml (as juice)

133.	*Cordia dichotoma* Forst. f. (*C. wallichii* G.Don)		
	Fruit	Shlashmotaka / Lisora / gondra	10-20 g
134.	*Cordia rotthii* Roem. and Schult. (Now known as *C. gharaf* (Forssk.) Ehrenb and Asch.		
	Fruit	Chhota Lisora / Lasudi	10-20 g
135.	*Coriandrum sativum* L.		
	Fruit / Seed	Dhanyaka / Dhaniya	1-3 g (as powder)
	Aerial part / Fresh leaf	Dhaniya	10-20 ml (as juice)
136.	*Costus speciosus / C. koeniga* (syn)		
	Rhizome / Root	Kebuka / Kemuk	2-4 g (as powder) (Not recommended for children below 5 years)
137.	*Crataeva nurvala* Buch- ham / *C. megna* DC		
	Fruit/Bark/Leaf	Varun / Barana	10-20 g (for decoction)
138.	*Crocus sativus* L.		
	Style/ Stigma	Kumkum (Kesar)	25-50 mg (Not recommended for children below 16 years)

139.	*Cucumis melo* L. / *C. melo* L. var. *momordica* Duthie and Fuller / *C. melo* L. var. *utilissimus* (Roxb.) Duthie and Fuller		
	Fruit	Kharbooja	50-100 g
	Seed		1-3 g (as powder)
140.	*Cucumis sativus* L.		
	Seed	Tripasha / Khira/cucumber	3-6 g (as powder)
	Fruit	Khira	50-100 g (as fresh)
141.	*Cucurbita maxima* Duch. ex Lam.		
	Seed	Peetkushmand/ Kashiphal/ kaddu	5 -10 g
	Fruit	Kashiphal	50-100 g (as fresh)
142.	*Cucurbita pepo* L.		
	Fruit	Kushmand / Safed Kaddu / safed petha	50-100 g (as fresh)
	Seed	Safed petha	5-10 g (as powder)
143.	*Cuminum cyminum* L.		
	Fruit	Jeerak / Jeera / safed	1-3 g (as powder)
144.	*Curculigo orchioides* Gaertn.		
	Tuber	Talmuli / Kalimushli	3-5 g

145.	*Curcuma amada* Roxb.		
	Rhizome	Aamra haridra / Ambaahaldi	5-10 g (as fresh) 2-4 g (as powder)
146.	*Curcuma angustifolia*		
	Root	Tavakasheer/ Tavkshir / Tikhur	2-5 g
147.	*Curcuma longa* L.		
	Rhizome	Haldi	1-3 g (as powder)
	Fresh Rhizome / Leaf		5-10 ml (as juice)
148.	*Curcuma zedoaria* Roxb. (Now known as *C. aromatica* Salisb.)		
	Rhizome	Karchura / Kachur	1-3 g (as powder)
149.	*Cyamopsis tetragonoloba*		
	Pod/Seed Gum	Gaurphali /Guar / Guar gum	20-30 g (as powder) 5-10 g (as powder)
150.	*Cymbopogon citratus*(DC.) Stapf / *C. coloratus*Stapf / *C. jwarankusa* (Jones) Schult / *C. martini* (Roxb.)Wats		
	Whole plant	Lamajjaka / Harichaya / Rosha Ghas / lemon grass	1-3 g (as infusion)
151.	*Cynodon dactylon* (L.) Pers.		
	Leaf / Whole plant	Durva / Duba	3-5 g

152.	*Cyperus rotundus* L. / *C. seariosus* R. Br		
	Rhizome	Mushtaka / Nagarmotha / Bhadramushtaka	2-5 g
153.	*Daucus carota* L.		
	Tuberous root	Gajar	50-100 g (as fresh) 50-100 ml (as juice)
	Seed		1-2 g (as powder) (Not recommended during pregnancy)
154.	*Desmodium gangeticum / D. latifolium*		
	Whole plant / Root	Shaalparnii / Sarvan	5-10 g (for decoction) 2-5 g (as powder)
155.	*Dillenia indica* L.		
	Fleshy fresh sepals / Bark / Leaf Fruit	Bhavya /Chalta	10-20 g (for decoction) 40-50 g (as fresh)
156.	*Dioscorea alata* L. / *D. deltoidea*		
	Tuber / Aerial bulbs	Kathalu / Shingali	10-20 g
	Extract		0.5-1 g

157.	*Dioscorea bulbifera* L.		
	Tuber /Aerial bulbs	Varahikand / Genthi / Taradi	20-30 g (as fresh) 5-10 g (as powder)
	Extract		0.5-1 g
158.	*Dioscorea esculenta* (Lour.) Burkill / *D. pentaphyla* L		
	Tuber	Madhvaluk / Suthani	5-10 g
159.	*Diplezia maxima*		
	Tender shoots	Lungru	30-50 g
	Root		5 – 10 g
160.	*Diospyros peregrina* Gurke (Now known as *D. malabarica* (Desr.) Kostel)		
	Ripe fruit	Tinduka / Tendu / Gab	20-30 g
	Unripe fruit	Gab	4-8 g (as powder)
	Bark / Leaf / Seed		3-5 g (as powder)
161.	*Dluchea lameolata C.B. Clarke*		
	Aerial parts / Leaf	Razana / Vaaya-surai	5-10 g (as powder)
162.	*Dolichos biflorus* L. (Now known as *Vigna unguiculata* (L.) Walp.)		
	Seed	Kulath / Kulathi Gontha	20-30 g

163.	*Dolichos lablab* L. (Now known as *Lablab purpureus* (L.) Sweet)		
	Seed	Nishpaav/ Sem/ Semphali	20-40 g (as seed)
	Tender Pod	Sem	30-40 g (as fresh)
164.	*Echinochloa frumentacea* Link / *Panicum frumentacea* (syn)		
	Fruit	Sanwa / Shyamaka	30-50 g
165.	*Eclipta prostata* L. / *E. alba* (syn)		
	Whole plant	Bhringaraj/ Bhangra	3-6 g (as powder)
166.	*Elettaria cardamomum* (L.) Maton		
	Seed	Elaa/ Sukshma elaa/ Chhoti elaichi	250-500 mg (as powder)
167.	*Eleusine coracana* (L.) Gaertn. ssp. *coracana* (Finger millet)		
	Seed	Madhuli / Madua / Ragi	20-50 g
168.	*Elsholtzia cristata* Willd. / *E. ciliate* (syn)		
	Leaf Seed	Ajogandha	5-10 ml (as juice) 2-3 g
169.	*Emblica officinalis* Gaertn. (Now known as *Phyllanthus emblica* L.)		
	Fruit	Amalaki/ Anwala / Amla	20-30 g (as fresh) 3-6 g (as powder) 5-10 ml (as juice)
	Extract		1-3 g

170.	*Embelia ribes* Burm. f.		
	Fruit	Vidanga / Vai-vidanga / Bhabhiranga	1-2 g (Not recommended for females planning to conceive)
171.	*Embelica tsjeriam* -cotton A.DC / E. robusta (syn)		
	Fruit	Vidanga (bhed) / Bai-vidang (bhed)	5-10 g (as powder)
172.	*Enicostemma littorale* Blume		
	Whole plant Extract	Maamajaka / Mamejwa / Naai	2-3 g 0.5 – 1 g
173.	*Ephedra gerardiana* Wall.		
	Leaf/Whole plant	Somlata / Som / Somvalli	2-3 g (as powder)
174.	*Euphorbia hidra* Linn. / *E. thymifolis* Linn.		
	Whole plant	Dugdhika / Dudhi	3-5 g (as powder)

175.	*Euphorbia neriifolia/ E. pilosa / E. royalana / E. dracunculoides*		
	Stem (tender) after boiling Leaf Latex	Snuhi / Thuhar / Sehund	10-20 g (as fresh) 3-5 g (as fresh) (Not recommended for children below 5 years and pregnant women) 20 – 30 mg
176.	*Euryale ferox* Salisb.		
	Seed	Makhana / Fox-nut	20-30 g (as seed) 3-5 g (as powder)
177.	*Fagopyrum esculentum* Moench. / *F. tataricum* Gaertn. / *F. essence*		
	Seed	Kuttu	30 -50 g
178.	*Ferula asafoetida* L. / Syn. *F. foetida* Regal/ F. narthex. Boiss		
	Oleo-gum resin	Hingu / Hing / Heeng	60- 125 mg (as powder)
179.	*Ficus benghalensis* L.		
	Fruit Shoot / Bark / Aerial root	Vatt / Nyagrodha / Baragad	40-50 g 5-10 g (for decoction) 2-5 g (as powder)

180.	*Ficus carica* L. / *F. palmata*		
	Fruit Leaf / Bark	Anjeer / fig / phalguni / Indian fig	20-30 g 3 – 5 g (as powder)
181.	*Ficus glomerata* Roxb. (Now known as *F. racemosa* L.)		
	Fruit / Leaf Bark	Udumbara / Gular	20-30 g (as fresh) 3 – 5 g (as powder)
182.	*Ficus hispida* L.f.		
	Fruit Bark	Kathgulara / Kakodumba	10-20 g 3 – 5 g (as powder)
	Tender leaf	Kathgulara	20-40 ml (as juice)
183.	*Ficus locar* Buch. Ham / *F. infectoria*		
	Fruit / Stem / Bark / Leaf	Plaksha / Pakad	5-10 g
184.	*Ficus religiosa* L.		
	Fruit / Tender Leaf	Aswath /Pipal / Peepal	5-10 g
	Bark		3 – 5 g (as powder)
185.	*Flacourtia ramontchi* L' Herit (Now known as *F. indica* (Burm.f.) Merr.) / *F. jangomas* (Lour.) Raeusch		
	Fruit	Vikantaka / Katai / Kanghu /Surva vruksha	5-10 g

186.	*Foeniculum vulgare* Mill.		
	Fruit Leaf	Mishraya / Sounf / Fennel seed	3-6 g (as powder) 20-30 g (as fresh)
187.	*Fumaria vaillantii* (Lois.) Hook. f. and Thoms. var. *indica* Haussk. (Now known as *F. indica* (Haussk.) Pugsley) / *F. parviflora* (syn)		
	Whole plant	Parpat / Pittapapda	1-3 g (as powder)
188.	*Garcinia indica* (Thour.) Choisy / *G. cambogia*		
	Mature fruit Butter/ Oil	Vrukshamala / Kokam	10-20 ml (as juice) 5-10 g (as powder) 3-5 g/ml
	Extract		1 – 2 g
189.	*Garcinia pedunculata* Roxb. ex Buch-Ham.		
	Fruit rind	Vatasamla / Amalbeda	5-10 ml/g (as juice/powder)
190.	*Gardenia gummifera* Linn. F		
	Gum	Naadihingu / Dikkamaali	250 – 500 mg
191.	*Gardenia turgida* Roxb. (Now known as *Ceriscoides turgida* (Roxb.) Tirveng.)		
	Gum	Kharahara / Mahapindi / Kharahatta	1-3 g (as powder)

192.	*Gentiana kurroo* Royle.		
	Rhizome / Root	Trayamana / Trayanta	1 – 3 g
193.	*Gisekia pharnaceoides* L.		
	Leaf	Elavallukavari / Baluka Saga	5-10 g
194.	*Glycine max* (L.) Merr.		
	Seed	Soya / Soyabean	20-40 g
	Soya proteins		10-20 g
195.	*Glycyrrhiza glabra* L.		
	Root / Stolon	Madhuyasti / Yashtimadhu / Mulethi / liquorice	5-10 g (as powder)
196.	*Gloriosa superba* Linn.		
	Root / Tubers	Langali / Kalihari	125 – 250 mg (not indicated in children and divine mothers)
197.	*Gmelina arborea* Roxb. / *Premna arborea* Roth (syn)		
	Fruit	Gambhari / Gamhari / Kaashmari	20-30 g
	Stem /Bark / Leaf		3 – 5 g (as powder)

198.	*Gmelina asiatica* L.		
	Fruit	Gopabhadra, Badhara	20-30 g
	Stem / Bark / Leaf		1 – 3 g (as powder)
199.	*Gossypium herbaceum / G. arboreum* L.		
	Seed Root	Karpasi/ Kapas/ Cotton	10-20 g 3 – 6 g (as powder)
200.	*Grewia hirsuta* Vahl		
	Root / Stem	Nagabala / Gulsakari	5-10 g (as powder)
	Fruit		3- 5 g
201.	*Grewia populifolia* Vahl (Now known as *G. tenax* (Forssk.) Fiori)		
	Bark / Fruit	Gangeru / Gangeran	5-10 g (as powder)
202.	*Grewia tiliaefolia* Vahl / G. sclerophylla / *G. optiva*		
	Fruit	Dhanvana / Dhamin	20-30 g
	Bark		3 – 5 g powder
203.	*Gymnema sylvestre* B. Br.		
	Plant	Meshashrungi / Gudmar / Madhunashini	5-10 g (for decoction) 3-5 g (as powder)
	Extract	Gudmar	0.5-1 g

204.	*Gynandropsis gynandra* (L.) Briq. (Now known as *Cleome gynandra* L.) / *G. pentaphyla* DC		
	Seed	Ajagandha / Hurhur	1-3 g (as powder)
	Whole plant	Hurhur	10-20 ml (as juice)
205.	*Habenaria intermedia / H. acuminata THW /H. edgeworthi*		
	Root tuber / Rhizome	Vruddhi / Ridhi	3-5 g
206.	*Hedychium spicatum* Ham ex Smith / *H. album*		
	Rhizome	Shatti / Kapur-Kachari	3-5 g
207.	*Helicteres isora* Linn.		
	Pod (fruit) / Bark / Leaf	Avartani / Avartaki / Marodphali	3-6 g (as powder)
208.	*Heliotropium indicum* Linn.		
	Whole plant	Hastishundi / Vrisehikaali	3-6 g (as powder)
209.	*Hemidesmus indicus* syn. *Periploca indicus* L.		
	Root / Stem	Anantmula	3-6 g
210.	*Hibiscus rosasinensis* L.		
	Flower	Japakusum/ Gudahal	1-3 g (as powder) (Not recommended during pregnancy)

211.	*Hibiscus sabdariffa* L.		
	Leaf	Abaasthaki/ Patawa	5-10 g (as powder)
	Seed	Patawa	1-3 g (as powder)
	Ripe calyx		5-10 g (as powder)
212.	*Hippophae rhamnoides* L. / *H. salicifolia*		
	Fruit / Leaf	Amlavetasa / Leh-beri/ Chharma/ Sea buck thorn	10-20 g
	Extract	Amalvets	0.5-2 g
213.	*Hordeum vulgare* L.		
	Seed	Yava/Jau	30-50 g
	Aerial parts (processed)/Ash		2-5 g
214.	*Hygrophila spinose / H. auriculata* syn. */ H. schull* (ham)		
	Seed *Whole plant*	Kokilaksha/ Ikshura / Tal makhana	3 – 6 g 1 – 3 g (as ash)
215.	*Hypericum perforatum*		
	Leaf / Whole plant	Basant	3-6 g
	Plant extract		0.5-1 g

216.	*Hyssopus officinalis* Linn.		
	Whole plant	Zuufea dayaa-kunji	3-5 g
217.	*Illicium verum* Hook. f.		
	Fruit	Badiyan Khatai /Aniseed star	250 - 500 mg (as powder)
218.	*Inula racemosa*. Hook / *I. roylanna* non- DC (syn)		
	Root	Pushkar mool / Pokhar mool	1-3 g (as powder)
219.	*Ipomoea aquatica* Forssk. / *I. raptans* por (syn)		
	Leaf	Kalambi / Kalamisaag	20-30 g
220.	*Ipomoea batatas* (L.) Lam.		
	Tuber	Shakarkandi / Mukhaalwka / Sweet potato	20-30 g
221.	*Ipomoea digitata* auct. non L. (Now known as *I. mauritiana* Jacq.)		
	Root/Tuber Seed	Kasheer – vidhara / Vidarikand	3-6 g 1-2 g
222.	*Ipomia nil* Linn. / *Convolvulus nil* Linn. / *Convolvulus biobatus* (syn)		
	Seed	Shankhini / Krishanbeej / Kaaladana	3-5 g (Not recommended in children below 5 years and pregnant women)

223.	*Juglans regia* Linn. / *J. cineraria* L.		
	Fruit/Endosperm Leaf/Bark	Akshod / Akhrot / Walnut	10-20 g 3-5 g
224.	*Juniperus communis*		
	Flower/Leaf	Hapusha / Hauber	2 – 6 g
225.	*Jusmin auriculata* Vahl. / *J. humile* Linn.		
	Leaf / Flower	Yuthika / Juhil / Swarn-yuthika (swarnjati)	3-5 g
226.	Jusmn *officinale* Linn. / *J. grandiflorum*		
	Leaf / Flower	Jaati / Chameli / Jasmin	3-5 g
227.	*Kaempferin galanga* Linn.		
	Rhizome	Sugandhvacha / Chandevmula	500mg – 1 g
228.	*Kigelia pinnata* Jaeg. DC .		
	Fruit Stem / Bark	Balam kheera	20-30 g 3-6 g
229.	*Lagenaria vulgaris* Ser. (Now known as *L. siceraria* (Mol.) Standl.)		
	Fresh fruit	Katutumbi / Tumbini	10-20 g
	Seed	Alabu	1-3 g (as powder)

230.	*Lagerstroemia indica / L. parviflora*		
	Leaf	Jarul	6 - 12 g (as powder)
	Extract	Frash/ Faransh	1-2 g
231.	*Lens culinaris* Medik.		
	Seed	Masura	20-40 g
232.	*Lepidium sativum* L.		
	Seed	Chandershoola / Chansur / Halon / Garden cress	3-6 g (as powder) (Not recommended during pregnancy)
	Aerial part	Chansur	30-50 g (as fresh)
233.	*Leptadenia reticulata* (Retz.)W. and A.		
	Leaf/ Aerial part Root / Whole plant	Jeevanti/ Dodisaka/ Hemavati	20-30 g (as fresh) 5-10 g (for decoction) 3-5 g (as powder)
234.	*Leucas cephalotus* (Koenig ex Roth) Spreng./ *L. aspera*		
	Leaf	Drona pushpi / Guma	20-30 g (as fresh) 3-5 g (as powder)

235.	*Limonia acidissima* L.		
	Fruit	Kapittha / Kainth / Wood apple	20- 40 g (as fruit)
	Leaf/Bark extract		1-3 g
236.	*Linum usitatissimum* L.		
	Seed	Alasi / Atasi/ linseed/flaxseed	10-20 g
	Seed oil	Atasi ka tail	10-20 ml
237.	*Litchi chinensis* Sonner		
	Fruit	Litchi	30-50 g
238.	*Luffa acutangula* (L.) Roxb.		
	Whole plant	Katu koshatakri / Torai / dhartorai / ridged gourd	5 -10 g (as powder)
	Fruit	Torai	30-50 g (as fresh)
	Seed		1-3 g (as powder)
239.	*Luffa cylindrica* (L.)M. Roem. / *L. echinata* (devdali)		
	Fruit	Dhaamargava /Nenua / Rajkoshataki	20-40 g (as fresh)
	Seed	Nenua	1-3 g (as powder)

240.	*Lycopersicon esculentum* Mill. (Now known as *L. lycopersicum* (L.) Karsten.)		
	Fruit	Tamatar/ tomato	20-40 g (as fresh)
241.	*Madhuca indica* Gmel.(Now known as *M. longifolia* (Koen.) Macbride var. / *M. longifolia* (Koenig) Macbride var. *latifolia*)		
	Flower	Madhuca / Mahua / jal mahua	10-15 g (as flower)
	Fruit	Mahua	10-15 g
	Seed oil	Koyna ka tail	2-5 ml
242.	*Malva sylvestris* L. / *M. rotundifolia*		
	Fruit	Suvarchala / Khubharaji / Gulkhair	5-7 g (as powder)
	Leaf	Gulkhair	3-6 g (as powder)
243.	*Mangifera indica* L.		
	Ripe fruit	Aamar / Aam	50-150 g
	Unripe fruit pulp	Aam	10-30 g
	Seed kernel	Aam Beej / Majja	1-2 g (as powder)
	Leaf / Bark	Aam	3-5 g
	Extract of leaf	*Amara (ghan)*	0.5-1 g
244.	*Maranta arundinacea* L.		
	Rhizome	Kookaineer (Sidha)/ Ararota/ Arrow-root	10-30 g (as powder)

245.	*Marrubium vulgare* Linn.		
	Whole plant	Fasaasiyum	3-5 g (as powder)
246.	*Marsilea minuta* L.		
	Leaf / Whole plant	Sunishannak/ Chowpatia	10-20 g (as fresh) 2-4 g (as powder)
	Extract	Chowpatia	0.5-1 g
247.	*Mentha spicata* L. / *M. arvensis* L. / *M. aquatica* Linn./ *M. suaveolans*		
	Aerial part	Putina/ Pudina	3-5 g
248.	Mentha *piperata* L./ *Mentha spp.*		
	Leaf	Peppermint / Sat pudina	2-5 g (as fresh) 1-2 g (as dry)
	Distilled oil/Extract		10-30 mg
249.	*Mesua ferrea* Linn.		
	Stemen/Flower bud	Nagkesar	1-3 g
250.	*Microstylis musifera* Ridley		
	Tuber	Jivaka	3-5 g
251.	*Microstylis wallichii* Lindl. (Now known as *Malaxis acuminate* D. Don)		
	Tuber	Rishabhka	5-10 g
252.	*Mimosa pudica*		
	Whole plant/Seed	Lajjalu / Lajwanti	3-6 g

253.	*Mimusops elengi* L.		
	Pericarp	Bakula / Maulsiri	20-40 g
	Flower	Maulsiri	5-10 g
	Bark		3-5 g
254.	*Mimusops hexandra* Roxb. (Now known as *Manilkara hexandra* (Roxb.) Dub.)		
	Pericarp	Khirni	20-40 g
255.	*Momordica charantia* L.		
	Fresh fruit / seed Dried fruit / seed Extract	Karabelwa / Karela	30-50 g (as fresh) 3-5 g (as seed) 0.5-1 g (Not recommended for females planning to conceive and children below 5 years)
256.	*Momordica dioica* Roxb. ex Willd.		
	Root	Karkotaka / Khekhasa/ Karkoda	3-6 g (as powder)
	Fruit	Khekhasa	30-50 g
257.	*Monochoria vaginalis* (Burm.f.)Presl.		
	Rhizome	Indivara	3-6 g

258.	*Moringa oleifera* Lam. / *M. concanensis* Nimmo		
	Leaf	Shiguru/ Sahijan / Muringya / Lal sehanjan	10-20 g (as fresh or paste) 2-5 g (as powder)
	Seed	Sahijan / Muringya	2-6 g (as fresh)
	Pod		40-80 g (as fresh) 2-5 g (as powder)
	Flower		10-20 g (as fresh)
	Extract of Bark/ Leaf/Fruit		0.5-1 g
259.	*Morus alba* L. / *M. Indica / M. nigra*		
	Fruit Tender leaf / Bark / Flower	Shahtoot / Toot	20-30 g 3-5 g
260.	*Morchella esculenta/M. elata*		
	Fruiting body	Guchhi	10-20 g

261.	*Mucuna pruriens* (L.) DC. / *M. prurita* Honk.		
	Root	Atma Gupta / Kapikachhu /	10-20 g (for
		Kawach/ Concha	decoction after processing)
	Pod	Kawach	20-30 g (as fresh after processing)
	Seed		3-6 g
	Extract		0.5-1 g
262.	*Murraya koenigii* (L.) Spreng. / *M. exotica* Linn (Kamini)		
	Leaf / Fruit	Kaidarya /meetha neem/ Kadhipatta	5-10 g
263.	*Musa paradisiaca* L.		
	Flower	Kadali / Kela / banana / plantain	20-30 g
	Fresh shoot	Kela	20-50 g 10-20 ml (as juice)
	Ripe Fruit		30-50 g
	Unripe Fruit		10-20 g
264.	*Myrica esculenta* Buch. Ham. / *M. nagi* Hook		
	Fruit	Kataphala / Kaiphal	5-10 g
	Bark	Kaiphal	2-3 g

265.	*Myristica fragrans* Houtt.		
	Seed (kernel)	Jatiphala / Jaiphala / Jatipatra	0.25- 1.0 g (Caution: excessive use may cause giddiness)
	Aril (outer part of fruit)	Javitri	0.25 -1 g (as powder)
266.	*Myristica malabarica* Lam.		
	Seed	Pashika / Pashupati / Jangali Jayaphala	0.5 -2 g
	Aril	Jangali javitri	0.25 -1 g
267.	*Nardostachys jatamansi* DC / *N. grandiflora*		
	Stem/Aerial parts *Extract*	Jatamansi / mansi	2-5 g 0.25-0.50 g
268.	*Nasturtium officinale/ N. aquaticum*		
	Leaf	Chhu-nalli / Water-cress / Piriya - haalim	10-20 g

269.	*Nelumbo nucifera* Gaertn.		
	Flower	Kamal / Padam	3-6 g (as powder)
	Rhizome	Bhen / Bhain	30-50 g (as fresh)
	Stalk	Murar / Kamalgatta	30-50 g (as fresh)
	Seed	kamalbeej	3-6 g (as powder)
270.	*Nymphaea alba* Linn/ *N. rubra*/ *N. stellate*		
	Rhizome/ Seed	Kumud – utpala / Kamlini/ Nilofer /Shavet/ rakta / neel kamal	10-20 g
	Flower		3-6 g
271.	*Nigella sativa* L.		
	Seed	Kalaunji / Kaala jaaji	1-3 g (Not recommended during pregnancy)
272.	*Nilgirianthus ciliatus* (Nees) / *Strobilanthes ciliatus* (syn)		
	Fruit	Sehachara	3-5 g (as powder)
273.	*Nyctanthes arbortristis* L.		
	Flower	Parijat / Shephaali/ Harshringara	1-2 g
	Leaf / Seed	Harshringara	1-3 g

274.	*Ocimum basilicum* L. / *O. pilosum* Wild.		
	Leaf	Barbari /Bhavari Tulsi/ Niajboo	3-6 ml (as juice) 1-3 g (as powder)
	Seed Extract		125-250 mg 0.25-0.50 g
275.	*Ocimum gratissimum* L.		
	Leaf / Seed Extract	Vriddha tulasi / Ram Tulasi	1-3 g (as powder) 0.25-0.50 g
276.	*Ocimum sanctum* L. (Now known as *Ocimum tenuiflorum* L.)		
	Leaf	Tulasi / Surasa / vrinda	2-5 g
	Seed Extract	Tulasi	1-2 g 0.25-0.50 g
277.	*Olea europaea*		
	Seed Oil Leaf	Zaitoon / Jaitun	10-20 g 10 – 20 ml 3-5 g (as powder)
278.	*Onosma bracteatum*		
	Whole plant/Leaf	Gojihraa / Gaozabaan	5-10 g
279.	*Onosma hispidum/ O. echioides* Linn.		
	Root	Ratanjot	3-5 g

279.	*Onosma hispidum/ O. echioides* Linn.		
	Root	Ratanjot	3-5 g
280.	*Operculina turpethum / Ipomea turpethum* (syn)		
	Root/Seed	Trivrat / Nishoth	1-3 g (Not recommended for children below 5 years)
281.	*Ophiocordyceps sinensis* / *O. indica* D.Don		
	Whole plant	Keetjaadi	20-60 mg
282.	*Opuntia vulgaris / O. dillenii*		
	Ripe fruit	Nagphani / Chhiter thohar	10-20 g (as fresh)
283.	*Orchis latifolia* L. (Now known as *Dactylorhiza hategeria* (D. Don) Soo)		
	Tuber	Mynjataka / Salampanja / Salam-mishu	3-5 g (as powder)
284.	*Origanum majorana* L. / Majorana hostensis (syn)		
	Leaf	Marubaka / Marnaa	5-10 drops (as juice)

285.	*Oroxylum indicum*		
	Bark/Seed	Shyonok / Sonapatha / Talvarphali / Tataplang	5-10 g (for decoction) 3-5 g (as powder)
286.	*Oryza sativa* L.		
	Seed Root stock	Shali-tandul / Chawal - shali	50-100 g 10-20 g (for decoction)
287.	*Oxalis corniculata* L.		
	Leaf	Changeri / Chukraa / Tinpatia	5-10 ml (as juice)
288.	*Paederia foetida* Linn.		
	Whole Plant	Prasarini / Gandh Prasarini	5-10 g (for decoction)
289.	*Panax pseudo ginseng* Wall / *P. quinquefolium* Linn. / *P. schinseg* Knees.		
	Root	Laxmana	1-3 g (as powder)
290.	*Pandanus odoratissimus* L.f. / *P. facicularis* Linn.		
	Oil Flower	Kethaki / Koedaa/ Kewada	2-5 drops 2-5 g

291.	*Panicum miliaceum* L. (Millet)		
	Seed (grains)	Chinast / Cheenaa	50-100 g
292.	*Papaver somniferum* L.		
	Seed	Posta-daana / Khas-Khas	1-2 g (if taken regularly) 2-5 g (as powder – occasionally)
293.	*Parmelia perlata* (Huds) Ach.		
	Whole plant	Lichen / Shaileya / Shailpushp / Chhareela	3-5 g
294.	*Paspalum scrobiculatum* L. (Kodo millet)		
	Seed	Kodrava / Kodon/ Kodo	50-100 g
295.	*Pedalium murex Linn.*		
	Fruit	Brihat Gokshura Bada gokharu	5 – 10 g (for decoction) 3-5 g (as powder)
296.	*Pennisetum typhoideum* L. C. Rich. (Now known as *P. americanum* (L.) K. Schum.) (Millet)		
	Seed	Bajra	20-40 g

297.	*Peucedanum graveolens* (L.) Benth. and Hook.f		
	Seed	Shepu	1-3 g
298.	*Phaseolus aconitifolius* Jacq. (Now known as *Vigna aconitifolia* (Jacq.) Marechal)		
	Seed Whole plant	Makushtha / Moth -dal	20-50 g 3 – 6 g (as powder)
299.	*Phaseolus aureus* Roxb. (Now known as *Vigna radiata* (L.) Wilczek var. *radiata*)		
	Seed Whole plant	Jangali moong	20-50 g 3 – 6 g (as powder)
300.	*Phaseolus lunatus* L.		
	Pod	Sem	25-50 g (as pulse)
301.	*Phaseolus mungo* L. (Now known as *Vigna mungo* (L.) Hepper)		
	Seed	Masha / Urad - kale	20-50 g (as pulse)
302.	*Phaseolus radiatus* L. / *P. trilobus* Sensu.		
	Seed	Mudga / Mudgaparni / Moong	50-100 g (as pulse)
303.	*Phaseolus vulgaris* L. / *P. namus* Linn.		
	Pod / Seed	Lobia / Rajma / Kidney bean	10-20 g (as pulse)

304.	*Phoenix dactilifera* L.		
	Fruit	Kharjuura / Khajur / Chuhara	20-30 g
305.	*Phoenix sylvestris* (L.) Roxb. / *P. acaulis*		
	Fruit	Kharjuura/ Khajoor –jungli	20-30 g
	Nira (Sap)	Khajoor	30-50 ml (as fresh juice)
306.	*Phyllanthus amarus / P. urinaria / P. fraternus* Webster		
	Plant	Tamlaki / Bhumyamalaki/ Bhui - amla	5-10 g
	Extract	Tamlaki	0.5-1 g
307.	*Physalis alkekengi* L.		
	Fruit	Raajabutraka / Winter cherry / Kaknaj	5-10 g
308.	*Physalis minima* L.		
	Fruit	Tankaari / Papoto	10-20 g

309.	*Physalis peruviana* L.		
	Fruit	Parpoti (var) / Rasbhari	10-20 g
310.	*Picorhiza kurroa* Royle Ex. Benth / P. *scrophularii* flora		
	Root	Katuk / Kutaki / Kulaki (Bheda)	1-3 g (as powder)
	Extract		125-250 mg
311.	*Pimpinella anisum* L.		
	Fruit	Anisoon / Aniseed	1-3 g
	Oil		0.5 - 1 ml
312.	*Pinus excelsa* / *P. wallichiana* (syn)		
	Fruit Oil Bark	Kail / Saral (var)	5-10 g 1-2 ml 2 – 3 g (Not recommended for children below 5 years)
313.	*Pinus gerardiana* Wall.		
	Endosperm Oil Bark	Nikochaka / Chilgoja / Neerachail	10-20 g 1- 2 ml 2 -3 g

314.	*Pinus roxburghii /P. longifolia Roxb*		
	Fruit / Oleoresin Oil	Saral / Cheer / Cheel	10-20 g 1-2 g 1-2 ml (Not recommended
			for children below 5 years)
315.	*Piper betle* L.		
	Leaf	Tambula / Pana-patta / Paan	2-5 g (Not recommended for children below 5 years)
316.	*Piper chaba* Hunter (non Blume) (Now known as *P.r retrofractum* Vahl)/ *P. officinarum*		
	Leaf	Chabya / Chabh / Chavika	1-3 g (as powder)
317.	*Piper cubeba* L.f.		
	Fruit	Kankola / Kabab chini	1-3 g (as powder)

318.	*Piper longum* L. / *P. retrofractum* Linn.		
	Fruit	Pippaali / Long pepper / Magha	0.5-2 g (as powder) (Not recommended for prolonged use)
319.	*Piper nigrum* L.		
	Fruit	Maricha / Kali Maricha/ Black pepper	0.5-2 g
320.	*Pistacia integerrima* Stewart (Now known as *P. chinensis* Bunge ssp. *integerrima* (Stewart) Rech.f.		
	Gall	Karkatasharingi / Kakadasingi / kakdain	1-2 g
321.	*Pistacia lentiscum* Linn.		
	Gum-Resin	Mastagi / Roomi-mastagi	2-3 g
322.	*Pistacia vera* L.		
	Seed endosperm	Mukuulaka / Pista	5-10 g
323.	*Pisum sativum* L.		
	Seed and pod	Matar	30-50 g (as fresh)

324.	*Plantago ovata* Forssk. / *P. major* Linn. / *P. lanceolata* Linn.		
	Seed Husk	Isabgol	5-10 g 5 – 10 g
325.	*Plumbago zeylanica* Linn. / *P. indica*		
	Root	Chitraka / Chitra-sfed / Lal-pushp	1-2 g (as powder) after purification (Not recommended for children below 5 years and pregnant women)
326.	*Podophyllum hexandrum* Poyle. / *P.emodii* Wall. (syn)		
	Fruit / Rhizome / Root	Ban-kakadi / Giriparpat	125-250 mg (Not recommended for children below 5
			years and pregnant women)
327.	*Pongania pinnorta* Pierre. / *P. glabra* syn		
	Seed Leaf/ Stem/ Bark Oil	Karanj	1-3 g (as powder) 3-5 g 1-2ml
328.	*Polygonatum cirrhifolium* (Wall.) Royle		
	Rhizome	Meda	5-10 g

329.	*Polygonatum verticillatum* (L.) All.		
	Rhizome	Mahameda	5-10 g
330.	*Portulaca oleracea* L. / *P. quadrifida* L.		
	Aerial part	Kulpha - sag / Nonia - sag	20-30 g (as fresh)
331.	*Premna integrifolia / P. latifolia / P. tomentosa*		
	Whole plant / Bark / Leaf	Agnimanth	5-10 g (as powder)
332.	*Prosopis spicegera* Linn. / *P.cineriaria* Druce/ *P. stephanianna* (syn)		
	Pods Leaf / Bark /Flower	Shami / Khekjjadii	Pods 20-30 g (as fresh) 3-6 g (as powder)
333.	*Prunus amygdalus* Baill. var. *dulchin*		
	Fruit seed	Vaataama / Badam	10-20 g
	Seed oil	Badam ka tail	3 - 5 ml
334.	*Prunus armeniaca* L.		
	Pericarp	Khumani / Aaluka / Apricot	10-20 g
	Kernel	Khumani	3-5 g
	Seed oil		3-5 ml

335.	*Prunus cerasoides* D. Dons / *P. puddum* Roxb. (syn)		
	Wood Flower	Padmaka / Padamkasht / Pajja/ Wild Himalaya cherry	1-3 g (as powder) 1 -2 g
336.	*Prunus domestika* Linn. / *P. communis* Huds.		
	Fruit Seed Oil	Aarak/ Aaluuchar / Aaluubhukaara	5-10 g (as dried fruit) 2-3 ml
337.	*Prunus persica* (L.) Batsch. / *P. vulgaris* Nutt.		
	Pericarp / Fruit	Aarun / Adu/ Aaluka/ Aru-adu	10-20 g
338.	*Psidium guajava* L.		
	Fruit	Peruka / Peru/ Amruda	20-50 g
	Leaf	Amruda	3-5 g

339.	*Pterocarpus marsupium* Roxb.		
	Heart wood	Asana /	5-10 g
	Extract	Vijaysar / Beejaka - beeja	0.5-1 g
340.	*Pterocarpus santalinus Linn.*		
	Heart wood	Rakt Chandan/ Lal chandan	5-10 g
341.	*Pterospermum cerifolium* Willd.		
	Flower Leaf	Muchukund	3-6 g 5-10 g
342.	*Pueraria tuberosa* (Roxb. ex Willd.) DC.		
	Tuber	Vidaari / Patal Kohda / Bhumi-kushmand / Lasood	10-20 g
343.	*Punica granatum* L.		
	Seed	Dadima/ Dadaka/ Anar	20-50 g
	Fruit rind	Anar	5-10 g
	Leaf		5 -10 g (for decoction)

344.	*Putranjiva roxburghii*		
	Fruit seed kernel	Putrajivak / Jiya-pota	3-6 g (Not recommended for children below 5 years)
345.	*Pyrus communis* L.		
	Fruit Seed Leaf	Nashpaati / Babbughosha	50-100 g 1 – 3 g 1-5 g (for decoction)
346.	*Pyrus malus* L. (Now known as *Malus pumila* Mill.)		
	Fruit	Seb	100-200 g 20-40 ml (as juice)
347.	*Ranunculus scleratus* Linn.		
	Whole plant /Root	Kaandir / Jal dhaniya	1-3 g (as powder)
348.	*Raphanus sativus* L.		
	Root / Leaf	Muulika / Muli	20-50 g (as fresh)
	Seed		125-250 mg
349.	*Reinwardtia indica*		
	Whole plant/Leaf Extract	Basanti	5-10 g (as powder) 0.5-1 g

350.	*Rhododendron arboreum* Sm. / *R. companulatum* / *R. lepidotum* Wall.		
	Flower	Rodo / Burans / Baraha	10-20 g
	Extract	Burans	1-2 g
351.	*Rheum emodi* Wall. ex Meissn. / *R. officinale*		
	Leaf Root / Stem	Revand chini / Peatmuli	0.5-1 g 1 – 2 g
352.	*Rhus parviflora* Roxb. ex DC. / *R. coriaria* Linn.		
	Fruit	Tinda / Samakdana	30-75 g
353.	*Ricinus communis*		
	Seed/ Root Leaf Oil	Erand / Arand / Castor seed	5-10 g 5-10 ml (as juice) 1-5 ml (as laxative occassionally) (Not recommended for children below 5 years)
354.	*Rosa alba* L. / *R. centifolia* L. / *R. damascena* Mill.		
	Flower Oil (distilled)	Gulab / Taaruni	10-20 g 2 – 5 drops

355.	*Roscoea procera* Wall.		
	Root tuber	Kakoli / Kandamula / Ksheerakakoli	5-10 g (as powder)
356.	*Rubia cordifolia*		
	Root/Stem	Manjishta / Manjeeth	1-2 g
357.	*Rumex vesicarius* L. / *R. nepalensis* / *R. maritimus* / *R. acetosella*		
	Leaf	Ambat chukka / Chukra	10-20 g (Not recommended for children below 5 years)
358.	*Saccharum Munja* Roxb. / *S. spontaneum* Linn.		
	Root	Shara-munja / Kaasha	10-20 g (for decoction) 6-10 g (as powder)
359.	*Saccharum officinarum* L.		
	Stem - Juice Root	Iiksashu/ Ganna	100-200 ml (as juice) 5-15 g (for decoction) (Not recommended for diabetics)

	Sugar	Chini / Shakkar	15-30 g (Not recommended for diabetics)
	Jaggery	Gud	15-30 g (Not recommended for diabetics)
360.	*Salacia chinensis* L. / *Salacia oblonga* Wall. ex Wight and Arn / *Salacia reticulata* Wight. / *S. roxburghii / S. macrosperma*		
	Root /Stem	Saptachakra / Saptrangi / Suvarnamula / Anakoranti ke mula	5-10 g (for decoction)
	Extract of root or stem	Saptrangi	0.5-1 g
361.	*Salix alba* Linn./*S. babylonical S. capral S. frag*. Lis / *S. tetraspermi*		
	Leaf / Bark / Root	Jalavetas / vetas / Bed-Mushak	10-20 g (for decoction) 3-6 g (as powder)
362.	*Salvadora persica/ S. oleoides*		
	Fruit/Leaf	Peelu / Bada pelu	5-10 g

363.	*Salvia aegiptica* Linn. / *S. moorcrafliana* / *S. officinalis*		
	Seed Plant	Tukhm-malanga / sage	1-2 g 3-5 g (as leaf powder)
364.	*Santalum album* L.		
	Oil	Chandan ka tail	3-5 drops
	Hard wood		1-2 g (as powder)
365.	*Saraca asoca Roxb.* / *S. indica*		
	Bark/Leaf	Ashok	5-10 g (Not recommended for children below 5 years)
366.	*Saussurea lappa* (Deeni) / *S. costus*		
	Root/Rhizome Oil	Kushta / Kuth	3-5 g (Not recommended for children below 5 years) 5-10 drops
367.	*Scindapsus officinalis* (Schoft)		
	Stem	Gajapipplai/ Gaj pippali / Gaj krishna	3-5 g

368.	*Scirpus kysoor* Roxb. (Now known as *S. grossus* (L.f.) Palla) / *S. tuberosus* Desf.		
	Rhizome Tuber	Kasheruk / Kasheru / Rajkasheruka	20-50 g (as fresh)
369.	*Selinum tenuifolium / S. vaginatum / S. Monnieri* Linn.		
	Rhizome /Root	Murra-Maangi / Bhuutakoshi	1-3 g
370.	*Semicarpus anacardium* Linn.		
	Fruits / Nuts	Bhallataka / Bhallava	Detoxified fruit 1-2 g in milk confection (Not recommdeded for children beow 5 years and pregnant women)
371.	*Sesamum indicum* L. (Now known as *S. orientale* L.)		
	Seed	Tila / Sesame / Gingelly	10-20 g
	Oil	Tila	5-10 ml
	Whole plant		2-3 g (as ash)

372.	*Sesbania grandiflora* (L.) Poir. / *S. susben* Linn.		
	Flower	Agasthya / Jayanti / Agathi / Jait	10-20 g (as fresh)
	Leaf	Agathi	10-20 g
373.	*Setaria italica* (L.) P. Beauv. (Millet)		
	Seed	Kanguni / Kangu	10-50 g
374.	*Shoria robusta* Gaertn.		
	Raisin Fruit / Bark /Wood Oil	Saala / Shaala	1-3 g 3-5 g (as powder) 1-3 ml
375.	*Sida cordifolia* L. / *S. rhombifolis* Linn./ *S. acuta* / *S. spinosel S. veronica* folia		
	Whole plant Extract	Balla / Mahaballa / Nagaballa / Rajaballa / Bariyara	10-20 g (for decoction) 1-2 g
	Seed	Bariyara	1-2 g

376.	*Sisimbrium rio* Linn./*S. losetii* Linn.		
	Seed Plant	Khuub Kalan	1-3 g 3-6 g (as powder)
377.	*Smilax china* Linn./*S. glabra* Roxb./ *S. lanceifolia* Roxb.		
	Tuber	Chobachini / Deepanter Vaacha	60-125 mg (as powder)
378.	*Solanum indicum / S. surattense / S. torvum / S. trilobetum* Linn.		
	Whole plant/ Root / Fruit	Bruhati / Kantkari-shavet	5-10 g (for decoction)
	Extract	Kateli	0.5-1 g
379.	*Solanum nigrum* L.		
	Whole Plant	Kakamachi / Chhoti Makoy / Mako	10-20 g
380.	*Sorghum vulgare* Pers. (Millet)		
	Seed	Jwara / Yaava - naal	50-100 g
381.	*Sphaeranthus indicus*		
	Flower	Mundi / Mundika / Gorakmundi	5-10 g

382.	*Spinacia oleracea* L.		
	Leaf	Palak / Spinach	30 -50 g
383.	*Spondias mangifera* Willd. (Now known as *S. pinnata* (L.f.) Kurz.)		
	Fruit Leaf / Bark	Aamrataka / Ambada / Kapitania	20-30 g 5-10 g (for decoction) 1-3 g (as powder)
384.	*Stephania glabra* Miers.		
	Tuber / Rhizome / Leaf	Raaja paatha / Kitha-kanehar	1-3 g (as powder)
385.	*Strychnos potatorum* L.		
	Seed	Kataki /	1-3 g (as powder)
		Nirmali	
386.	*Swertia chirayita / S. ciliata / S. angustifolia*		
	Whole plant	Kiratik / Cheretta / Bhuunimba / Chiraita	3-5 g
	Extract	Chiraita	0.5-1 g

387.	*Symplocos racemose Roxb. / S. paniculata* Thunb.		
	Bark/Leaf	Lodhara / Lodhera - pathani	3-5 g
388.	*Syzygium aromaticum* (L.)Merr. and L.Perry		
	Flower bud	Lavanga / Laung	0.5-1 g
389.	*Syzygium cuminii* (L.) Skeels		
	Pericarp and mesocarp	Jambu / Jamun	10-50 g
	Seed	Jamun	3-5 g
390.	*Tacca aspera* Roxb.		
	Tuber	Bhevara ke kand	20-30 g
391.	*Tamarindus indica* L. / *T. officinalis* Hk (syn)		
	Fruit pulp	Amlika / Chincha / Imali / Tamarind	2-5 g (Not recommended during skin ailments)
	Seed	Imali	5-10 g
392.	*Taraxacum officinale*		
	Leaf /Whole Plant	Dugdh - pheni / Dudhi / Dandelion	1-2g (as powder)

393.	*Taxus baccata*		
	Leaf Bark	Talis patra/ Sthavneyak / Thunera / Birmi	1-3 g (as powder) 3-5 g (as powder)
394.	*Tecomella undulata* Seem.		
	Bark	Rohitaka / Roheda	15-30 g (for decoction) 3-6 g (as powder)
395.	*Tephrosia purpurea*		
	Whole plant	Sarponkha	5-10 g (for decoction) 3-5 g (as powder)
396.	*Teramnus labialis* (L.f.) Spreng.		
	Whole plant	Mashaparni	10-20 g (for decoction)
397.	*Terminalia arjuna Roxb.*		
	Bark/Leaf/Fruit	Arjun / Parth	1-5 g
	Extract	Arjun	0.5 -1 g

398.	*Terminalia belerica* (Gaertn.) Roxb.		
	Fruit pericarp	Bibitaki Bahera	3-5 g
	Extract	Bahera	0.5-1 g
399.	*Terminalia catappa* L.		
	Kernel	Jungali badaama / Desi badama	10-20 g
400.	*Terminalia chebula* Retz.		
	Fruit pericarp	Haritaki / Harad / Shiva	3-5 g (as powder)
	Extract	Harar	0.5-1 g
401.	*Terminalia tomentosa* Wight. and Arn.		
	Stem/Bark/Leaf	Asana / Jarandrum / Asan	5-10 g (for decoction) 3-5 g (as powder)
402.	*Tetragonia expansal T. tetragonoides* Pall.		
	Shoots / Seed / Root / Flower	Van-paalak	20-50 g (as fresh) 5-10 g (as powder)
403.	*Thalictrum foliolosum* DC.		
	Plant / Root	Peetranga / Mamirii	1-2 g (as powder)

404.	*Thespesia populnea* soland.		
	Stem / Bark	Paarisha / kapitana / Paarish-pippala	10-20 g (for decoction) 3-6 g (as powder)
405.	*Thymus serpyllum* auct. non L. (Now known as *T. linearis* Benth.) / *T. vulgaris*		
	Leaf	Banya-ajwain / Ban ajwain	1-3 g (as powder)
406.	*Tilia cordata* Linn. / *T. Vulgaris*		
	Flower	Telia	2-5 g (as powder)
407.	*Trachyspermum ammi* (L.) Sprague		
	Seed	Yavani / Ajwain / Desi ajwain	1-3 g (as powder)
	Leaf	Ajwain	3 -5 g
	Oil		5-10 drop
408.	*Trapa bispinosa* Roxb. (Now known as *T. natans* L. var. *bispinosa* (Roxb.) Makino)		
	Endosperm / Fruit	Shrungataka / Singhada / Sigadu	30-60 g
409.	*Trianthema portulacastrum* L.		
	Whole plant	Varsha vhun / Vishakhaparna	1-3 g

410.	*Tribulus terrestris* Linn.		
	Fruit/Whole plant	Gokhru / Gokshura	2-4 g (as powder) 5-10 g (for decoction)
411.	*Tricholepis glaberrima* DC.		
	Plant	Brahmadandi / Brahm dandi	3-6 g
412.	*Trichosanthes anguina* L.		
	Fruit	Dadhipushpi / Chichinda	30-60 g
413.	*Trichosanthes dioica* Roxb.		
	Fruit/ Leaf	Patola /	10-20 g
		Parawal	
414.	*Trigonella foenum-graceum* L.		
	Seed	Methika / Methi	1-2 g (soaked in water or germinated or roasted)
	Leaf	Methi	50-100 g (as fresh)
415.	*Triticum aestivum* L.		
	Seed	Gehun	50-100 g
	Tender shoot/spout	Ankurita Gehu	10-30 g

416.	*Typhonium trilobatum* (L.) Schott.		
	Tuber	Karu karunai / Konchu	20-50 g
417.	*Tinospora cardifolia* Miers. (Menispermaceae) syn. *T. glabra* (n. Burm) / *T. crispa* Linn.		
	Roots/Stem	Guduchi / Amrita-valli / Giloya / Giloy	5-10 g (as powder) 10-20 ml (for decoction) 0.5-1 g Max (as sattva)
	Extract		0.5-1 g
418.	*Trichosanthes bracteata* Lam. / *T. palmata* Roxb. (syn)		
	Root / Fruit	Inder Vaaruni / Vishaalaa	0.5-1 g (as powder) (Not recommended for children below 5 years and pregnant women)
419.	*Urtica parviflora / U. dioica*		
	Tender Leaf	Vrishchhiya – shaakiar / Bicchubuti	10-20 g (for decoction)

420.	*Uraria picta / U. crinita* Desv / *U. pililifera* Linn.		
	Whole plant	Prishnaparni Pithvin	5-10 g (for decoction) 3-5 g (as powder)
421.	*Urginea indica* Roxb. Kunth / *Drimia indica* Roxb. (syn)		
	Bulb / Root / Leaf	Van palandu / jangali piyaz / kolakand	125-250 mg (Not recommended for children below 5 years and pregnant women)
422.	*Valeriana jatamansi* Jones / *V. wallichii*		
	Rhizome	Sugandh –baalaa / Tagar	1-3 g (as powder)
423.	*Veronika officinalis* / *V. teres* Wall.		
	Whole plant / Leaf	pamukha	0.25 – 1 g
424.	Vetiveria zizanioides		
	Whole plant	Ushira / Khas / Vetiver	5 - 10 g (for decoction)
425.	*Vigna trilobata* (L.) Verdc.		
	Whole plant	Mudadaparni / Mugvan	2-4 g (as powder)

426.	*Viola odorata / V. pilosa / V. sylvestris*		
	Whole plant Flower	Banafsha / Vanksha	3-5 g 1-2 g
427.	*Vitex agnus-castus* Linn.		
	Seed Leaf	Renuka beej / Sage	1-2 g 1-3 g (Not recommended for children below 5 years)
428.	*Vitex negundo / V. trifolia*		
	Fruit/Seed/Leaf	Nirgundi / Sambhaalu	1-3 g
429.	*Vitis vinifera* L.		
	Fruit dry	Draksha / Munakka	5-10 g
	Seed / Fruit skin	Munakka	1-3 g
430.	*Wedelia calendulacea* (L.) Less. (Now known as *W. chinensis* (Osbeck) Mer.)/ *W. biflora* DC.		
	Leaf	Peet-bhringraja/ Pila bhagra	5-10 g (for decoction) 1-3 g (as powder)

431.	*Withania coagulans* (Stocks) Dunal		
	Fruit	Desi – asgandh / Paneer doda	3-10 g
432.	*Withania somnifera* (L.) Dunal.		
	Root	Ashwagandha / Asgandh / Nagauri / asgandha	3-6 g (as powder)
	Extract	Asgandh	0.5-1 g
433.	*Woodfordia fruticosa*		
	Flower	Dhataki pushp / Dhay ke phool	3-5 g
434.	*Wrightia tinctoria / W. tomentosa*		
	Bark/Leaf Seed	Svet kutaj / Meetha kutaj / Inderyava	3- 5 g 1-3 g
435.	*Zanthoxylum alatum* Roxb. (Now known as *Zanthoxylum armatum* DC.)		
	Seed / Bark	Timura / Tejovati / Tis-mira	1-3 g
436.	*Zea mays* L.		
	Seed	Makka	20-50 g
	Anthers / Corn silk		3-5 g

437.	*Zingiber officinale* Rosc.		
	Rhizome	Adrakh / Shunti	5-10 g (as fresh) 1-3 g (as dried) 0.1 – 1 g (Not recommended during hypertension
	Extract		and bleeding disorders)
438.	*Zizyphus jujuba* Lam.		
	Pericarp	Unnaba / unnab ber	10-50 g (as fresh) 10-20 g (as powder)
439.	*Zizyphus nummularia* (Burm.f.) W. and A. / *Z. oenoplia* / *Z. xylopyra* Willd.		
	Pericarp	Jangali Ber / Jhar ber	15-30 g (as fresh fruit)
	Leaf		3-6 g (as powder)

Source: FSSAI

Note 1. Ingredients listed in the above Schedule shall be used after due processing or in their extract forms subject to permissible usage range given in the last column of the table. Offering these ingredients, either alone or in combinations as such or minimally processed (cleaned, de-weeded, sorted, dried or powdered) is/are not permitted.

Note 2. The ingredients listed above shall comply with Food Safety and Standards (Contaminants, Toxins and Residues) Regulations,2011.

Note 3. The permitted range of usage for children between 5-16 years is ½ of the permitted range of usage for adults.

Note 4. The permitted range of usage for children between 1-5 years is ¼ of the permitted range of usage for adults."

SCHEDULE – VI

List of Ingredients as Nutraceuticals

PART A				
Sl. No.	**Nutraceutical ingredients**	**Official/Common name**	**Purity Criteria**	**Permitted Range**
1.	American ginseng (*Panax quinquefolius* L.)	Ginseng extract (American).	American ginseng extract (Containing NLT 10% of total ginsenosides ondried basis).	90-400 mg/day, Max
2.	Astaxanthin (from *Haematococus pluvalis*), powder or oleoresin	-	Astaxanthin content	4 mg/day, Max
3.	Beta Alanine	-	-	4-6 g/day, Max (not more than 4 weeks at a stretch)
4.	Betaine (N,N,N,-tri-methylglycine)	-	-	600-650 mg/day, Max
5.	Boswellia serrata-gum resin extract	Salai guggul/Kundru	Total boswelic acids or 11-keto-beta boswelic acids content	250-1, 500 mg extract/ day, Max

[Table Contd.

Contd. Table]

Sl. No.	Nutraceutical ingredients	Official/Common name	Purity Criteria	Permitted Range
		PART A		
6.	Caffeine	Caffeine	Per cent caffeine	Within levels specified in FSS Regulations
7.	Calcium hydroxyl methyl butyrate	-	CaHMB content	3-6 g/day, Max (Not recommen-ded for use by pregnant women and lactating mothers)
8.	Chromium picolinate/ nicotinate	-	Chromium picolinate/ nicotinate content	200-400 mcg/day, Max
9.	*Cimicifuga racemosa* (*or Actaea racemosa*). Extracted from rhizomes and roots	Black cohosh	Total triterpene glycosides (minimum 0.4%), calculated as 23-epi-26-deoxyactein).	40-200 mg/day, Max
10.	Citrus bioflavonoids (*Citrus paradisi, C. reticulate, C.maxima, C. sinensis and Citrus limon*)	Citrus/Jambir	Bioflavinoids and total polyphenol content	150-600 mg/day, Max
11.	CoQ10 from non GM source	Co enzyme Q10	Ubiqinone and ubiqinol content	100-1,000 mg/day, Max

[Table Contd.

Contd. Table]

PART A				
Sl. No.	Nutraceutical ingredients	Official/Common name	Purity Criteria	Permitted Range
12.	Colostrum	-	-	Bovine colostrum spray driedpowder at usage level of 15g per day (containing 3g of IgG) or 3g per day (containing 0.3 g IgG) without any efficacy claims.
13.	Creatine	-	-	3 g/day, Max (for adults only)
14.	Cryptoxanthin/ Mesoxanthin	-	-	3 mg/day, Max
15.	Echinacea (*E. angustifolia, E. purpurea, and E. pallida*) *Liquid/powder extract*	Echinacea	Alkamides (0.25 mg/ml) and cichoric acid (2.5 mg/ml), if the extract used is in liquid form. In case of Hydroethanolic Echinacea extract is in a powdered form computation may be done proportionately to the weight/weight dry powder extract based on liquid extract used to obtain a dry powder format.	900 mg/day, Max

Table Contd.

Contd. Table]

PART A

Sl. No.	Nutraceutical ingredients	Official/Common name	Purity Criteria	Permitted Range
16.	Ginkgo biloba extract obtained from dried leaves of Ginkgo *(Ginkgo biloba. L.).*	Ginkgo biloba extract	Ginkgo flavone glycosides and Ginkgolides (diterpene lactones). Total flavonoids content (20.2 to 27% calculated as flavanol glycosides and tested for total terpene lactones (5.4% to 12.0%). Presence of Ginkgolides A, B, C needs to be testedqualitatively.	120-240 mg/day, Max
17.	Glucosamine hydrochloride	Glucosamine	Glucosamine content	1,500-3,000 mg/day, Max
18.	Glucosamine sulphate	Glucosamine	Glucosamine content	2,500-5,000 mg/day, Max
19.	Glutathione	-	-	50 mg-600mg/day, Max
20.	*Gymnema sylvestre* extract powder	Madhunashin i, Gudmar (extract)	Gymnemic acid content	500-1,500 mg/day, Max
21.	Lactase (β-galactosidase)*	-	Enzyme activity	3,000–9,000 IU (or FCCunits)/day,
22.	L-carnosine	-	-	130-600 mg/day, Max
23.	L- theanine	Chai suksham satva		50-100 mg/day, Max

Table Contd.

Contd. Table]

PART A

Sl. No.	Nutraceutical ingredients	Official/Common name	Purity Criteria	Permitted Range
24.	Melatonin	-	-	2–10 mg/day, Max
25.	Methyl sulfonyl methane	-	-	1000-3000 mg/day, Max (Not recommended for use by pregnant women and lactating mothers)
26.	*Panax ginseng* (Syn; Korean Ginseng) extract - (obtained from 0.6 to 2.0 g of Ginseng root, (*Panax ginseng*. C A. Meyer, Araliaceae)	Ginseng extract	Ginsenoside content ranging from 3-10% and adjusted to potency basis 3% total ginsenoside content	90-400 mg/day, Max
27.	Phycocynin from *Spirulina plantesis (Aethrospira plantesis)* Dried powder	Spirulina	Protein: 50-70 %; Carbohydrates: 20-40%; Minerals (Ash): 5.0–15%; Moisture: 3.0–6.0%	50–250 mg/day, Max
28.	*Piper nigrum/Piper longum* extract	Pippali/Pepper	Piperine content	15 mg/day of piperine, Max (Duration of use: maximum 30 days)

Table Contd.

Contd. Table]

PART A				
Sl. No.	Nutraceutical ingredients	Official/Common name	Purity Criteria	Permitted Range
29.	Quercetin obtained from extracts of citrus fruits and other vegetables	-	Quercetin content	100 mg/day, Max
30.	*Schizandra* berry extract	Five-flavor berry	Schizandrin berries containing 2.5-3.0% schizandrin	1–3 g/day, Max
31.	*Scutellaria bicalensis*	Patwar topi, Skullcap	Aq. Extract Standardized to bicallin content 30–50% and adjusted to potency basis 50% bicallin content	250–1,000 mg/day, Max
32.	Selenium Yeast	-	Selenium content and number of yeast counts (Cfu/g)	2 mg/day of selenium, Max
33.	Siberian ginseng-obtained from 0.6 to 2.0 g of Ginseng root (*Acanthopanax-senticosus*, belonging to panax type, C A. Meyer, Araliaceae)	Ginseng extract	Eleutherosides content	100–450 mg/day, Max

Table Contd.

Contd. Table]

PART A				
Sl. No.	**Nutraceutical ingredients**	**Official/Common name**	**Purity Criteria**	**Permitted Range**
34.	*Silybum marianum* extract (silymarin extract)	Milk Thistle	Standardized extract – silimarin content	250-1,000 mg/day, Max
35.	Spirulina (algae) from (*Spirulina platensis, Arthrospira platensis)*	Shaiwal/Spirulina	(Protein (min.) - 55%, carbohydrates (max.)- 30%, fats (lipid) – not more than 10%, minerals (ash)- 5-10%, moisture- 3-6% (also fatty acid profile to be mentioned on the package)	500-3,000 mg/day, Max
36.	Undenatured type II collagen	-	-	40 mg/day, Max
37.	*Vaccinium myrstillus* extract	*Bilberry extract*	Anthocyanin content	50-600 mg/day, Max
38.	Zeaxanthin			4 mg/day, Max

PART B		
Sl. No.	**Nutraceuticals/Ingredients**	**Official and Common Names**
1.	(+) Hydroxycitric acid	-
2.	*Albizia lebbeck* - extract	Shireesh
3.	*Allium sativum* – bulbs dried standardized powder/extract	Rason/Lashun/Garlic
4.	*Aloe vera* – juice/concentrate/powder of sap/gel	Ghrit Kumari/Indian aloe
5.	Alpha-amylase*	-
6.	Alpha mangostin	-
7.	Alpha-galactosidase*	-
8.	Alpha-lipoic acid	-
9.	*Amaranthus tricolor* – leaf powder/extract	Marisha-Rakt Extract
10.	Amylase*	-
11.	Amyloglucosidase*	-
12.	*Anethum graveolens* L. - seeds and oil	Shatahva/Sowa/Soa/Dill
13.	Anthocyanin	-
14.	Arabinogalactan	-
15.	Arachidonic acid	-
16.	*Asparagus densiflorus* - extract	Asparagus/Shatavari
17.	*Bacopa monnieri* - leaf extract	Brahmi
18.	Barley seed powder	Yava/Barley
19.	*Bauhinia variegata* - extract	Kachnar
20.	*Berberis vulgaris/B. aristata/B.asiatica* – stem/root extract	Berberry/Daru haridra
21.	Beta carotene – standardized soft concentrate/emulsified concentrate/ powder	-
22.	Beta ecdysterone	-
23.	β-glucans	-
24.	*Beta vulgaris* – root extract	Palanki/Beet

[Table Contd.

Contd. Table]

Sl. No.	Nutraceuticals/Ingredients	Official and Common Names
25.	β-sitosterol	-
26.	*Betula platyphylla/B.utilis* - bark extract	Bhojapatra/Birch
27.	*Biota orientalis* - seed powder	Biota
28.	*Camellia sinensis*-Black/green tea extract, standardized powder	Chai & tea extract
29.	*Borago officinalis* - oil	Borage
30.	Campestanol	-
31.	Campesterol	-
32.	*Capsicum annum* - extract/standardized to capsicin content	Lanka/Cayenne pepper/ Lal mirchi
33.	*Caricus papaya* – leaf extract	Papaya/Papeeta, Erand-karkati
34.	Carotenoids (natural mixed, including from algal sources)	-
35.	Casein and caseinates	-
36.	*Caulophyllum thalictroides* - root extract	Blue cohosh
37.	Cellulase*	-
38.	*Centella asiatica* – leaf/aerial parts standardized extract	Mandukparni/Gotu Kola
39.	*Matricaria chamomilla (Matricaria recutita*) – aerial parts extract	Chamomile
40.	*Malpighia emarginata* (Cherry acerola)	Acerola
41.	*Chlorella* ***vulgaris*** – dried powder	Green algae/Shaiwal
42.	Chlorogenic acids	-
43.	Caffeic acid	
44.	Chondroitin sulphate	Chondroitin
45.	*Cichorium intybus* – roasted root powder	Kasani/Chicory
46.	*Cinnamomum verum* – bark powder/extract	Tvak bhed/Cinnamon
47.	Citrulline	-

[Table Contd.

Contd. Table]

Sl. No.	Nutraceuticals/Ingredients	Official and Common Names
48.	*Citrus aurantium* – peel extract/ bioflavonoids standardized	Bitter orange
49.	Citrus naringenin	-
50.	D-Mannose	-
51.	*Syzygium aromaticum*- Clove powder & oil	Lavang tail
52.	*Cnicus benedictus* – aerial parts extract/ root extract	Blessed thistle
53.	*Theobroma cacao*-Cocoa (chocolate) bean - extract	-
54.	*Coccinia grandis* (L.) Voigt - extract	Bimbi/Kunduru/Ivy gourd
55.	Collagen and its hydrolysed peptides and chelates	-
56.	Conjugated linoleic acid concentrate	-
57.	*Crataeva nurvala* - extract	Varun
58.	Crustacean shells	-
59.	*Cuminum cyminum* L – oil/extract standardized	Jeerak/Safed Jeera/ Cumin
60.	*Curcuma longa* – rhizome powder/extract	Haridra/Haldi/Turmeric
61.	Curcuminoids – soft extract/powder and curcumin complex	-
62.	*Cyperus rotundus* - extract	Mustak/Nagar motha
63.	Dehydroepiandrosterone (DHEA) and 7-Keto DHEA	-
64.	Diastase*	-
65.	D-Pinitol	-
66.	*Dioscorea bulbifera* - extract	Varahi kand
67.	Edible legumes (seed powder), legume proteins (protein isolates/concentrates/ hydrolysates)	-

[Table Contd.

Contd. Table]

Sl. No.	Nutraceuticals/Ingredients	Official and Common Names
68.	Ellagic acid	-
69.	*Emblica officinalis* – dried fruit extract/ spray-dried pulp powder	Indian gooseberry/amlaki
70.	Eriocitrin (from citrus fruit)	-
71.	*Oenothera biennis*- Evening primrose oil	-
72.	*Fagopyrum esculentum* - seed	Buckwheat
73.	Fish oil	-
74.	*Foeniculum vulgare* - fruit - oil/extract	Fennel/Saunf
75.	Freeze-dried banana powder	-
76.	Galactomannan	-
77.	Gallic acid	-
78.	Gamma-linoleic acid (GLA)	-
79.	Gamma-oryzanol	-
80.	*Garcinia gummi-gutta and Garcinia cambogia/G.indica* – fruit rind extract standardized to hydroxyl citric acid,	Kokum/Vrikshamalak/ Malabar tamarind powder)
81.	*Garcinia mangostana* – seed extract standardized	Mangosteen
82.	Glucoamylase*	-
83.	Glucomannan	-
84.	*Glycyrrhiza glabra* - extract	Madhuyashti/Licorice/ Mulethi
85.	Grape seed extract	-
86.	*Coffea arabica, C. robusta*- Green coffee seed extract standardized, including decaffeinated coffee bean powder/extract	Kaphi
87.	*Grifola frondosa* – standardized extract	Maitake mushroom
88.	Guar gum and gum arabic and its derivatives as a source of fibres; and fibres from other food sources	Guarphali

[Table Contd.

Contd. Table]

Sl. No.	Nutraceuticals/Ingredients	Official and Common Names
89.	Hemicellulase*	-
90.	Hesperidin	-
91.	High oleic sunflower oil and other vegetable oils with high oleic content	-
92.	*Hippophae rhamnoides* – leaf/fruit dried powder/extract/juice	Amalvetas/Sea buckthorn/
93.	*Humulus lupulus* L – powder/extract	Perhaps/Hops
94.	Hyaluronic acid and its salts	-
95.	Hydrolysed whey peptide	Whey
96.	*Hypericum perforatum* – aerial parts standardized extract	Basant/St. Johns Wort
97.	*Inula racemosa* - root extract	Pushkarmoola extract
98.	Invertase*	-
99.	Isoflavones (genistein, daidzein)	-
100.	Kelp (brown algae)	-
101.	Krill oil - standardized for DHA/EPA	-
102.	Lactalbumin	-
103.	Lactoferrin	-
104.	Lactoperoxidase*	-
105.	*Lagerstroemia speciosa* L (leaf extract)	Jarul/Banaba
106.	Lecithins	-
107.	Lignans	-
108.	*Linum usitatissimum* - seed powder and oil	Atasi/Alasi/Flaxseed
109.	Lipase*	-
110.	Lutein	-
111.	Lutein/zeaxanthin complex	-
112.	Lycopene	-
113.	*Lycium elaeagnus* - fruit - dried powder/ concentrate standardized	Goji berry (wolfberry)

[Table Contd.

Contd. Table]

Sl. No.	Nutraceuticals/Ingredients	Official and Common Names
114.	Maltase*	-
115.	*Mangifera indica* – mangiferine, leaf extract	-
116.	*Medicago sativa* extract	Ashar-bala/Alfalfa
117.	Medium chain triglycerides	-
118.	*Menyanthes trifoliata* - Leaf powder	Buckbean/bogbean
119.	Millets and their powder	-
120.	*Momordica charantia* - fruit/seed extract	Karvalli/Kodon,/bitter gourd/,Karela
121.	*Monodora myristica* (Gaertn.) Dunal – oil/ extract	Nutmeg
122.	*Morinda citrifolia* extract	Akshiki/Noni
123.	*Moringa oleifera* leaf/pods/seed extract powder	Shigru/Moringa/drum stick
124.	*Morus alba*- Mulberry tea– leaf/fruit extract	Toot/Mulberry
125.	*Myrica cerifera/M. nagi* – bark extract	Katphala/Bayberry
126.	*Myristica fragrans Houtt.*	Jatipatri/Mace/Javitri
127.	N-Acetyl d-glucosamine	-
128.	*Nardostachys jatamansi* - extract	Jatamansi
129.	*Nasturtium officinale* - extract	Chhu nail/Watercress
130.	Nattokinase enzyme (as Soybean Fibrinase)	-
131.	*Ocimum tenuiflorum/Ocimum sanctum* – aerial parts/seed extract	Surasa/Basil/Tulasi
132.	Omega-3 fatty acids (docosahexaenoic acid - eicosapentaenoic acid - alpha-linolenic acid)	-
133.	Omega-6-fatty acids (linoleic acid, arachidonic acid and conjugated linoleic acid)	-
134.	Oyster shell powder	Shukti/Seep
135.	Pancreatin*	-

[Table Contd.

Contd. Table]

Sl. No.	Nutraceuticals/Ingredients	Official and Common Names
136.	Pancrelipase*	-
137.	Papain*	-
138.	*Passiflora foetida* - extract	Passion flower
139.	*Arachis hypogaea* - (roasted) powder	Mandapi/Pea nut/ Munghphali
140.	Pectin	-
141.	Pepsin*	-
142.	*Perna canaliculus* (Green-lipped mussel/ Mussel Oil)	-
143.	*Phellodendron amurense* leaf oil	Phellodendron
144.	Phosphatides/Phospholipids	-
145.	*Phyllanthus amarus* - extract	Tamalaki/Bhuiamalaki
146.	Phytase*	-
147.	*Picrorhiza kurroa*-Picrorhiza - extract	Katuka/Kutaki
148.	*Pimento officinalis* L. - extract/powder	Allspice
149.	*Pinus gerardiana* - bark extract	Nikochak/Pine nut
150.	*Piper longum* - extract	Pippali/Magha/Long pepper
151.	*Piper nigrum* - green extract	Green pepper, Krishan Marich
152.	*Piper nigrum*– powder/standardized extract	Krishan Marich/Marich/ Black pepper
153.	Policosanol	-
154.	Protease*	-
155.	*Prunus serotina* - extract	Black cherry
156.	*Plantago ovata* (major) –Psyllium (Isaphula)- seed husk	Isaphgul-Ashabgol
157.	*Cucurbita pepo, C. maxima*- Pumpkin seed oil/meal	Kaddu beej tail

[Table Contd.

Contd. Table]

Sl. No.	Nutraceuticals/Ingredients	Official and Common Names
158.	*Punica granatum* – fruit/seed/skin extract/ leaf/powder	Dadima/Pomegranate
159.	*Raphanus sativus var. niger* - root powder/ extract	Mulika/Muli/Black radish
160.	Red wine - extract/concentrate	-
161.	Red yeast rice	-
162.	Resveratrol	-
163.	*Rhododendron arboreum/R. campanulata* - juice/extract	Buras/Rhododendron
164.	Rice bran	-
165.	Rice bran arabinoxylan compound	-
166.	Rose hips	-
167.	*Rosmarinus officinalis* – leaves/needles extract/oil	Rosemary
168.	Royal Jelly	-
169.	Rutin from fruit peels	-
170.	*Salvia officinalis* – leaf extract	Renuka Leaf Extract/Sage
171.	*Sambucus nigra* - extract	Khaman Kabir/Elderberry/ Black elderberry
172.	Shark cartilage/squalene oil	-
173.	Shiitake mushroom - extract	-
174.	*Solanum lycopersicum/S. esculentum* – fruit powder/extract	Tamatar/Tomato
175.	Soy sprouts – dried powder	-
176.	Soya protein isolate/edible legume seed protein isolate	-
177.	Spearmint – leaf and distillate	-
178.	Sterols/Stanols including their esters and cholesterol	-
179.	*Tagetes sp.* – petals oleoresin/extract	Marigold

[Table Contd.

Contd. Table]

Sl. No.	Nutraceuticals/Ingredients	Official and Common Names
180.	*Camellia sinensis* - Tea catechins (epigallo catechin gallate, epicatechin, catechin gallates)	Chai satva
181.	*Terminalia arjuna* - bark/leaf extract (standardized extract)	Arjuna Ext.
182.	*Terminalia bellerica* - fruit extract	Bibhitak/Baheda/ Myrobalan
183.	*Terminalia chebulia* - fruit extract	Haritaki/Harad/Myrobalan
184.	Theaflavin	Chai sukshara satva
185.	Theobromine	-
186.	Tocopherols	-
187.	*Trigonella-foenum-graecum* – seeds extract	Methika/Methi/Fenugreek
188.	*Triticum sativum* - bran	Godhum/Wheat/Gehu
189.	Trypsin*	-
190.	*Vaccinium corymbosum* - fruit - dried powder/concentrate standardized	Blueberry
191.	*Vaccinium oxycoccos/Vaccinium macrocarpon* - fruit - dried powder/ concentrate standardized	Cranberry
192.	*Valeriana wallichii* - extract	Tagar
193.	*Vitis alba and Vitis vinifera* - fruit - dried powder/concentrate standardized	Draksha/Munakka/Blue grapes
194.	Wheat germ	-
195.	*Zingiber officinale* - standardized rhizome extracts	Shunti/Ginger

Note. - *Enzymes- The enzymes listed in this schedule are primarily used as processing aids, but also may be used in nutraceutical products.

Source: FSSAI

SCHEDULE - VII

List of strains as probiotics (live micro-organisms)

S. No.	Name of the Microorganism
1.	*Lactobacillus acidophilus*
2.	*Lactobacillus plantarum*
3.	*Lactobacillus reuteri*
4.	*Lactobacillus rhamnosus*
5.	*Lactobacillus salivarius*
6.	*Lactobacillus casei*
7.	*Lactobacillus brevis*
8.	*Lactobacillus johnsonii*
9.	*Lactobacillus delbrueckii* sub- sp. *bulgaricus*
10.	*Bacillus coagulans*
11.	*Lactobacillus fermentum*
12.	*Lactobacillus caucasicus*
13.	*Lactobacillus helveticus*
14.	*Lactobacillus lactis*
15.	*Lactobacillus amylovorus*
16.	*Lactobacillus gallinarum*
17.	*Lactobacillus delbrueckii*
18.	*Bifidobacterium bifidum*
19.	*Bifidobacterium lactis*
20.	*Bifidobacterium breve*
21.	*Bifidobacterium longum*
22.	*Bifidobacterium animalis*
23.	*Bifidobacterium infantis*
24.	*Streptococcus thermophilus*
25.	*Saccharomyces boulardii*
26.	*Saccharomyces cerevisiae*
27.	*Lactobacillus paracasei*

28.	*Lactobacillus gasseri*
29.	*Bacillus clausii*
30.	Established probiotic strains of *Bacillus subtilis*"

Source: FSSAI

Note. (1) These organisms may be used either singly or in combination but shall bedeclaredon the label with full information and has to beNon-GMO.

(2) The Food Autho3rity may add any new strain of microorganism, possessing probiotic properties, after proper scientific evaluation, and include in thisSchedule.

SCHEDULE - VIII

List of prebiotic compounds

S.No.	Prebiotic Compounds
1.	Polydextrose
2.	Soya poly-saccharides and Soybean oligosaccharides
3.	Isomalto-oligosaccharides
4.	Fructo-oligosaccharides
5.	Gluco-oligosaccharides
6.	Xylo-oligosaccharides
7.	Inulin
8.	Isomaltulose
9.	Genito-oligosaccharides
10.	Lactulose
11.	Lactoferrin
12.	Sugar alcohols such as lactitol, sorbitol, maltitol, inositol, isomalt
13.	Galacto-oligosaccharides

Source: FSSAI

REFERENCES

Adams, G. G.; Imran, S.; Wang, S.; Mohammad, A.; Kok, S.; Gray, D. A.; Channell, G. A.; Morris, G. A. and Harding, S. E. (2011). The hypoglycaemic effect of pumpkins as anti-diabetic and functional medicines. *Food Res. Int.*, **44**: 862-867.

Adams, P. B.; Lawson, S.; Sanigorski, A. and Sinclair, A. J. (1996). Arachidonic acid to eicosapentaenoic acid ratio in blood correlates positively with clinical symptoms of depression. *Lipids*, **31**(1): S157–S161.

Anonymus, (2016). Food Safety and Standards (Health Supplements, Nutraceuticals, Food for Special Dietary Use, Food for Special Medical Purpose, Functional Food and Novel Food) Regulations, 2016. Retrieved from the FSSAI website: https://fssai.gov.in/upload/uploadfiles/files/Nutraceuticals_Regulations.pdf.

Applequist, W. L.; Avula, B.; Schaneberg, B. T.; Wang, Y. H. and Khan, I. A. (2006). Comparative fatty acid content of seeds of four Cucurbita species grown in a common (shared) garden. *J. Food Compos. Anal.,* **19**: 606-611.

Arnoldi, A. (2010). Nutritional Pharmacy. Proceedings of the EAFP, Catania Symposium, June 24-26, 2010, Departmentio di Endocrinologia, Fisiopatologia e Biologia Applicata, University of Milano and HPF- Nutraceutics SRL.

Bagchi, D. (2006). Nutraceuticals and functional foods regulations in the United States and around the world. *Toxicol*, **221**: 1-3.

Barberan, T. H. and Robins, R. J. (1997). Phytochemistry of fruits and vegetables: Oxford Science Publication.

Barreca, D.; Laganà, G.; Leuzzi, U.; Smeriglio, A.; Trombetta, D. and Bellocco, E. (2016). Evaluation of the nutraceutical, antioxidant and cytoprotective properties of ripe pistachio (Pistacia vera L., variety Bronte) hulls. *Food Chem.*, **196**: 493-502.

Beceanu, D. (2008). Nutritive, nutraceutical, medicinal and energetic value of fruits and vegetables. *Cercetri Agronomice în Moldova.,* **4** (136): 65- 80.

Bell, S. J. and Goodrick, G. K. (2002). A Functional Food Product for the Management of Weight Critical Reviews in Food Science and Nutrition, **42**: 163-178.

Bickford, P. C.; Tan, J.; Shytle, R. D.; Sanberg, C. D.; El-Badri, N. and Sanberg, P. R. (2006). Nutraceuticals synergistically promote proliferation of human stem cells. *Stem Cells Dev.*, **15**: 118-23.

Bland, J. S. (1996). Phytonutrition, phytotherapy and phytopharmacology. *Altern.Ther. Health Med.*, **2**: 73-76.

Brouns, F. (2014). Soya isoflavones: a new and promising ingredient for the health foods sector. *Food Research International*, **35**: 187-193.

Burgo, L. S. Z.; Hernández, R. M.; Orive, G. and Pedraz, J. L. (2014). Nanotherapeutic approaches for brain cancer management. *Nanomed. Nanotech. Biol. Med.*, **10**: 905 919.

Burney, P. G.; Comstock, G. W. and Morris, J. S. (1989). Serologic precursors of cancer: serum micronutrients and the subsequent risk of pancreatic cancer. *Am. J. Clin. Nutr.,* **49**: 895–900.

Chahed, T.; Dhifi, W.; Hamrouni, I.; Msaada, K.; Bellila, A. E.; Kchouk, M. and Marzouk, B. (2007). Comparison of pistachio hull essential oils from different Tunisian localities. *Ital. J. Biochem.,* **56**, 35-39.

Chauhan, B.; Kumar, G.; Kalam, N. and Ansari, S. H. (2013). Current concepts and prospects of herbal Nutraceutical: A review. *J. Adv. Pharm. Technol. Res.*, 4(1): 4-8.

Das, L.; Bhaumik, E.; Raychaudhuri, U. and Chakraborty, R. (2012). Role of nutraceuticals in human health. *J. Food. Sci. Technol.,* **49**(2): 173.

DeFelice, S. L. (1995). The Nutraceutical Revolution: its impact on food industry. *Trends Food Sci. Technol.,* **6**: 59-61.

Dejica, D. (2001). *Antioxidanci _i terapie antioxidant.* Edit. Casa crcii de _tiinc, Cluj Napoca.

Devi, V. K. and Rehman F. (2002). Nutraceutical antioxidants- An overview. *Indian journal of Pharmaceutical Education,* **36**(1): 3-8.

Dulloo, A. G.; Duret, C. and Rohrer, D. (1999). Efficacy of a green tea extract rich in catechin polyphenols and caffeine in increasing 24-h energy expenditure and fat oxidation in humans. *Am. J. Clin. Nutr.*, **70**: 1040-1045.

Dumitrescu, C. (1987). *Bazele practicii alimentatiei dietetice profilactice si curative,* Edit. Medical, Bucure_ti.

El-Samaligy, M. S.; Afifi, N. N. and Mahmoud, E. A. (2006). Evaluation of hybrid liposomes encapsulated silymarin regarding physical stability and in vivo performance. *Int. J. Pharm.* **319**: 121-129.

Engelbrecht, A. M.; Mattheyse, M.; Ellis, B.; Loos, B.; Thomas, M.; Smith, R.; Peters, S.; Smith, C. and Myburgh, K. (2007). Proanthocyanidin from grape seeds inactivates the PI3 kinase/PKB pathway and induces apoptosis in a colon cancer cell line. *Cancer Lett.*, 258: 144-153.

Favier, L. C. et al., (1995). *Répertoire général des aliments.* Edit. Tec&Doc, Paris.

Feng, J. G. and Chen, L. Q. (2003). Determination of procyanidin in grape seed extracts. *China Food Addit.,* **6**: 103-105.

Florlani M. et al., 2003 – *Contenuto in sostanze ad attitivita antiossidante nelle pesche: variabilita indota da cultivar, stadio di maturazione e frigoconservazione*. Rev. Frutticoltura nr. 7-8

Frasher, P. D. (2006). Phytosterols as functional food components and Nutraceuticals. *Phytochemistry*, **67**: 212-214.

Freeman, M. P.; Hibbeln, J. R.; Wisner, K. L.; et al. (2006). Omega-3 fatty acids: evidence basis for treatment and future research in psychiatry. *Journal of Clinical Psychiatry*, **67**(12): 1954–1967.

Gibson, G. R. and Roberfroid, M. B. (1995). Dietary modulation of the human colonic microbiota: introducing the concept of prebiotics. *J. Nutr.*, **125**(6): 1401-1412.

Giovannucci, E. (2002). A review of epidemiologic studies of tomatoes, lycopene and prostate cancer. *Exp. Biol. Med.,* **227**: 852-859.

Goff, S. A. and Klee, H. J. (2006). Plant volatile compounds: Sensory clues for health and nutritional value? *Science,* **311**: 81- 819.

Goli, A. H.; Barzegar, M. and Sahari, M. A. (2005). Antioxidant activity and total phenolic compounds of pistachio (Pistacia vera) hull extracts. *Food Chem.,* **92**: 521-525.

Goncea, I. (1970). *Alimentacia* racional *a omului*, Edit. Didactic _i Pedagogic, Edit. Tehnic, Bucure_ti

González-Sarrías, A.; Larrosa, M.; García-Conesa, M. T.; Francisco, A.; Barberán, T. and Espín, J.C. (2013). Nutraceuticals for older people: Facts, fictions and gaps in knowledge. *Maturitas*, **75**: 313–334.

Hamid, A. A. and Luan, Y. S. (2000). Functional properties of dietary fiber prepared from defatted rice bran. *Food Chemistry*, **68**: 15-19.

Hamilton, M.; Gibson, G. R. and Bruck, W. (2003). Some insights into the derivation and early uses of the word 'probiotic'. *British Journal of Nutrition*, **90**: 845.

Hamilton-Miller, J. M. (2003). The role of probiotics in the treatment and prevention of Helicobacter pylori infection. *International Journal of Antimicrobial Agents,* **22**(4): 360-366.

Hibbeln, J. R. (1998). Fish consumption and major depression. *The Lancet*, **351**(9110): 1213. Horrobin, D. F. (1998) Schizophrenia: the illness that made us human. *Medical Hypotheses*, **5**(4): 269-288.

Hui, Y. H. F.; Chen, F. and Nollet, L. M. L. (2010). Handbook of Fruit and Vegetable Flavours. John Wiley & Sons, New Jersey, U.S.A.

Inti, M. and Faoro, F. (2006). Grape phytochemicals: a bouquet of old and new nutraceuticals for human health Medical Hypotheses, **67**: 833-838.

Jing, P.; Song, L. H.; Shen, S. Q.; Zhao, S. J.; Pang, J. and Qian, B. J. (2014). Characterisation of Phytochemicals and Antioxidant Activities of Red Radish Brines during Lactic Acid Fermentation. *Molecules*, **19**: 9675–9688.

Kalra, E. K. (2003). Nutraceutical-definition and introduction. *AAPS Pharm. Sci.*, **5**: 27-28.

Keservani, R. K. and Sharma, A. K. (2014). Flavonoids: emerging trends and potential health benefits. *Journal of Chinese Pharmaceutical Sciences*, **23**(12): 815–822.

Kimpel, F.; Schmitt, J. J. (2015). Review: Milk proteins as Nanocarrier systems for hydrophobic nutraceuticals. *J. Food Sci.*, **80**: R2361–R2366.

Lee, C. H.; Jeong, T. S.; Choi, Y. K.; Hyun, B. H.; Oh, G. T.; Kim, E. H.; Kim, J. R.; Han, J. I. and Bok, S. H. (2001). Anti-atherogenic effect of citrus flavonoids, naringin and naringenin, associated with hepatic ACAT and aortic VCAM-1 and MCP-1 in high cholesterol-fed rabbits. *Biochem. Biophys. Res. Commun.*, **284**: 681–688.

Lin, C. C.; Lin, H. Y.; Chi, M. H.; Shen, M. H.; Chen, H. W.; Yang, W. J. and Lee, M. H.(2014). Preparation of curcumin microemulsions with food-grade soybean oil or lecithin and their cytotoxicity on the HepG2 cell line. *Food Chem.*, **154**: 282–290.

Liu, R. H. (2003). Health benefits of fruit and vegetables are from additive and synergistic combinations of phytochemicals[1–4]. *Am. J. Clin. Nutr.*, **78** (suppl.): 517S.

Maswal, M. and Dar, A. A. (2013). Inhibition of citral degradation in an acidic aqueous environment by polyoxyethylene alkylether surfactants. *Food Chem.*, **138**: 23562364.

Matsufuji, H.; Kido, H.; Misawa, H.; Yaguchi, J.; Otsuki, T.; Chino, M.; Takeda, M. and Yamagata, K. (2007). Stability to light, heat, and hydrogen peroxide at different pH values and dpph radical scavenging activity of acylated anthocyanins from red radish extract. *J. Agric. Food Chem.*, **55**: 3692–3701.

McCann, J. C. and Ames, B. N. (2005). Is docosahexaenoic acid, an n-3 long-chain polyunsaturated fatty acid, required for development of normal brain function? An overview of evidence from cognitive and behavioral tests in humans and animals. *The American Journal of Clinical Nutrition*, **82**(2): 281-295.

McClements, D. J. (2010). Emulsion design to improve the delivery of functional lipophilic components. *Annu. Rev. Food Sci. Technol.,* **1**: 241–269.

Mermel, Vl. (2004). Old paths new directions: use of functional foods in the treatment of obesity. *Trends in Food Science and Technology*, **15**: 532-540.

Muniraj, I. K.; Xiao, L.; Liu, H. and Zhan, X. (2015). Utilisation of potato processing waste water for microbial lipids and linolenic acid production by oleaginous fungi. *J. Sci. Food Agric.,* **95**: 3084–3090.

Nordvisk, E.; Salomonsson, A. C. and Aman, P. (1984). Distribution of insoluble bound phenolic acids in barley grains. *J. Sci. Food. Agric.*, **35**: 657-661.

Okamoto, T. (2005). Safety of quercetin for clinical application (Review). *Int. J. Mol. Med.* **16**: 275-278.

Olinescu R. et al., 1990 – *Mecanisme de aprare a organismului împotriva polurii chimice.* Edit. Tehnic, Bucure_ti

Pandey, M.; Verma, R. K. and Saraf, S. A. (2010). Nutraceuticals: new era of medicine and health. *Asian J, Pharm. Clin. Res.,* **3**: 11-15.

Peet, M.; Laugharne, J. D. E.; Mellor, J. and Ramchand, C. N. (1996). Essential fatty acid deficiency in erythrocyte membranes from chronic schizophrenic patients, and the clinical effects of dietary supplementation, *Prostaglandins Leukotrienes and Essential Fatty Acids*, **55**(1-2): 71–75.

Peppelenbosch, M. P. and Ferreira, C. V. (2009). Immunology of pre and probiotic supplementation. *Br. J. Nutr.,* **101**: 2-4.

Picard Marie-Amélie, 2008– *Alimentacia preventiv împotriva cancerului.* Edit. Polirom, Ia_i

Proust Ingrid, 2008 – *Des raisins plus riches en antioxydants.* Rev. Réussir Fruits et Légumes, nr. 269

Rahman, M. M.; Ichiyanagi, T.; Komiyama, T.; Hatano, Y. and Konishi, T. (2006). Superoxide radical and peroxynitrite-scavenging activity of anthocyanins; structure-activity relationship and their synergism. *Free Radic. Res.,* **40**: 993-1002.

Rai, S. P.; Pandey, N.; Meena, R. P. and Rai, S. K. (2011). A Review Article on Medicinal Plants Derived Nutraceuticals: A Re- Emerging Health Aid. *International Journal of Pharma and Bio Sciences,* **2**(4): 419– 437.

Rajaei, A.; Barzegar, M.; Mobarez, A. M.; Sahari, M. A. and Esfahani, Z. H. (2010). Antioxidant, anti-microbial and antimutagenicity activities of pistachio (Pistacia vera) green hull extract. *Food Chem. Toxicol.,* **48**: 107-112.

Rajasekaran, A.; Sivagnanam, G. and Xavier, R. (2008). Nutraceuticals as therapeutic agents: A Review. *Res. J. Phar. Technol.,* **1**: 328-340.

Ramaa, C. S.; Shirode, A. R.; Mundada, A. S. and Kadam, V. J. (2006). Nutraceuticals an emerging era in the treatment and prevention of cardiovascular diseases. *Curr. Pharm. Biotechnol.,* **7**: 15-23.

Ravi Subbiah, M. T. (2007). Nutrigenetics and Nutraceuticals: the next wave riding on personalised medicine. *Translational Research.,* **149**: 55-61.

Sagar, B. P. S.; Zafar, R.; Tyagi, K.; Kumar, V.; Kumar, S. and Panwar, R. (2004). 'Antioxidants', The Indian Pharmacist, 29-35.

Sano, T.; Oda, E.; Yamashita, T.; Naemura, A.; Ijiri, Y.; Yamakoshi, J. and Yamamoto, J. (2005). Antithrombotic effect of proanthocyanidin, a purified ingredient of grape seed. *Thromb. Res.,* **115**: 115-121.

Schieber, A.; Stintzing, F. C. and Carle, A. (2001). By-products of plant food processing as a source of functional compounds- Recent developments. *Trends Food Sci. Technol.,* **1**: 401-413.

Segal B. et al., 1986 – *Factori de proteccie prezenci în produsele alimentare.* Edit. Junimea, Ia_i

Segal, R.; Segal. B. *et al.*, (1983) *Valoarea nutritiv a produselor agroalimentare.* Edit. Ceres, Bucure_ti.

Shena, L. N.; Zhanga, Y. T.; Wang, Q.; Xub, L. and Fenga, N. P. (2014). Enhanced in vitro and in vivo skin deposition of apigenin delivered using ethosomes. *Int. J. Pharm.,* **460**: 280-288.

Shrikhande, A. (2000). Wine by-products with health benefits. *Food Res. Int.* **33**: 469-474.

Shukla, Y. and Singh, M. (2007). Cancer preventive properties of ginger: a brief review. *Food and Chemical Toxicology,* **45**: 683-690.

Sirtori, C. R. and Galli, C. (2002). Fatty acids and the Omega-3. *Biomedecine and Pharmacotherapy.,* **56**: 397-406.

Slimestad, R.; Fossen, T. and Vagen, I. M. (2007). Onions: A source of unique dietary flavonoids. *J. Agric. Food Chem.,* **55**: 10067-10080.

Soong, Y. Y. and Barlow, P. J. Antioxidant activity and phenolic content of selected fruit seeds. *Food Chem.,* **88**: 411-417.

Spranger, I.; Sun, B.; Mateus, A. M.; Freitas, V. and Ricardo-da-Silva, J. M. (2008). Chemical characterisation and antioxidant activities of oligomeric and polymeric procyanidin fractions from grape seeds. *Food Chem.*, **108**: 519-532.

Takahashi, M.; Uechi, S.; Takara, K.; Asikin, Y. and Wada, K. (2009). Evaluation of an oral carrier system in rats: Bioavailability and antioxidant properties of liposome-encapsulated curcumin. *J. Agric. Food Chem.,* **57**: 9141–9146.

Tavano, L.; Muzzalupo, R.; Picci, N. and Cindio, B. (2014). Coencapsulation of antioxidants into niosomal carriers: Gastrointestinal release studies for nutraceutical applications. *Colloids Surfaces B Biointerfaces,* **114**: 82-88.

Tucker, G. (2003). Nutritional enhancement of plants. *Current Opinion in Biotechnology*, **14**: 221-225.

Varzakas, T.; Zakynthinos, G. and Verpoort, F. (2016). A Review on Plant Food Residues as a Source of Nutraceuticals and Functional Foods. *Foods J.*, **5**: 88.

Vattem, D. A. and Shetty, K. (2005). Biological Function of Ellagic Acid: A Review. *Journal of Food Biochemistry,* **29**(3): 234-266.

Wargovich, M. J. (2000). Anticancer properties of fruits and vegetables. *Hort. Science,* **35**: 573-575.

Whitman, M. (2001). Understanding the perceived need for complementary and alternative Nutraceuticals: lifestyle issues. *Clin. J. Oncol. Nurs.,* **5**: 190-94.

Wilkerson, T. M.; Weaver, L.; Hovius, C. and Zandstra, J. W. (2007). Nutritional and Health Benefits of Fresh Vegetables – Past, Present and Future: A Literature Review. CORD IV Project # 9021 Final Report, 7.

Wu, A.; Ying. Z and Gomez-Pinilla, F. (2007). Omega-3 fatty acids supplementation restores mechanisms that maintain brain homeostasis in traumatic brain injury. *Journal of Neurotrauma*, **24**(10): 1587-1595.

Yoo, J.; Baskaran, R. and Yoo, B. (2013). Self-nanoemulsifying drug delivery system of lutein: Physicochemical properties and effect on bioavailability of warfarin. *Biomol. Ther.*, **21**: 173-179.